VETERINARY SCIENCES AND MEDICINE

INNOVATIVE ETHNO VETERINARY PRACTICES IN THE CONTROL OF NEWCASTLE DISEASE AND HELMINTHOSIS IN POULTRY IN SOUTH WESTERN UGANDA

VETERINARY SCIENCES AND MEDICINE

Additional books in this series can be found on Nova's website under the Series tab.

Additional e-books in this series can be found on Nova's website under the e-book tab.

VETERINARY SCIENCES AND MEDICINE

INNOVATIVE ETHNO VETERINARY PRACTICES IN THE CONTROL OF NEWCASTLE DISEASE AND HELMINTHOSIS IN POULTRY IN SOUTH WESTERN UGANDA

CHARLES LAGU
AND
FREDERICK I. B KAYANJA

nova publishers
New York

Library of Congress Cataloging-in-Publication Data

Innovative ethno veterinary practices in the control of Newcastle disease and helminthosis in poultry in south western Uganda / Charles Lagu and Frederick I.B. Kayanja (Biology Department, Faculty of Science, Mbarara University of Science and Technology, Mbarara, Uganda), editors.
pages cm. -- (Veterinary sciences and medicine)
Includes bibliographical references and index.
ISBN 978-1-63117-299-1 (hardcover)
1. Poultry--Virus diseases--Uganda. 2. Newcastle disease--Uganda. 3. Poultry--Parasites--Uganda. 4. Veterinary epidemiology--Uganda. I. Lagu, Charles, editor. II. Kayanja, F. I. B., editor.
SF995.6.V55I56 2015
636.5'0896096761--dc23
2014040994

Published by Nova Science Publishers, Inc. † New York

We dedicate this work to small, medium, large scale and organic Poultry farmers in the world

CONTENTS

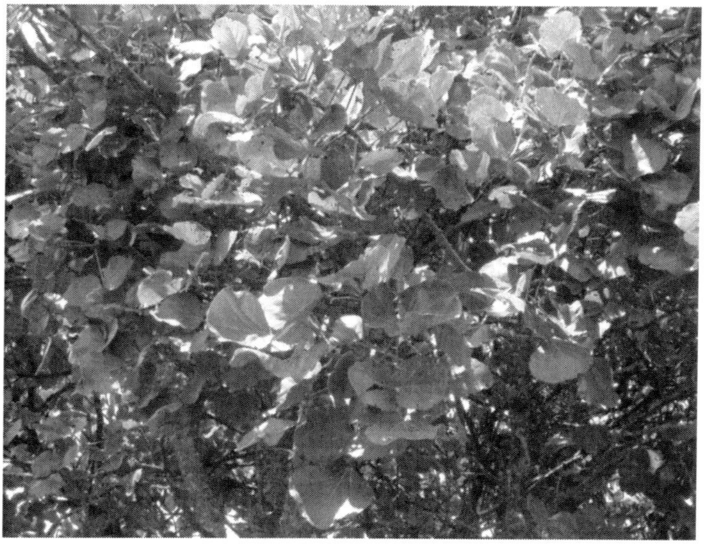

Erythrina abyssinica Lam.ex DC plant

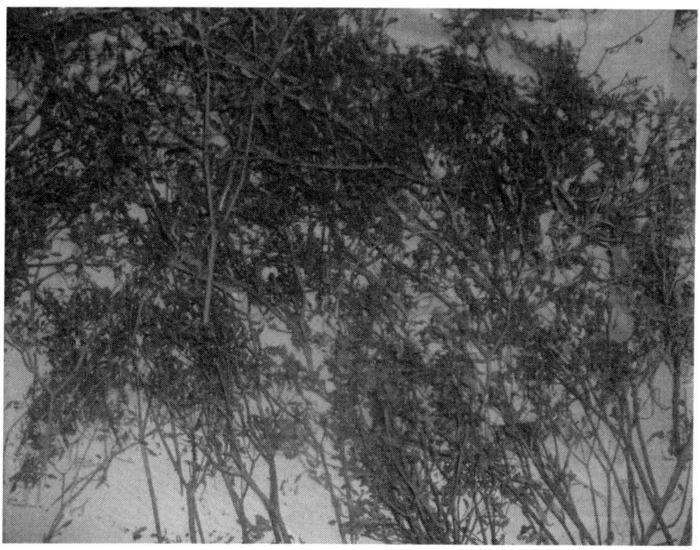

Capsicum annum L plant.

SEPTEMBER, 2014

DECLARATION

We declare that the information contained in this book is our original piece of work except where the contributions of others are acknowledged. We declare that the work has not been submitted in any form to any other research institution or publishing house/publisher.

ACKNOWLEDGMENTS

Gratitude goes to Belgian embassy in Uganda through the Belgian Technical Cooperation for supporting the research work at Mbarara University of Science and Technology (MUST) for the past three years. This facilitation came at a crucial time when resources were scarce.

Dr. Eunice Olet is thanked for her role in botanical identification of the plants species *Capsicum annum* and *Erythrina abyssinica* and also for reviewing the book. The contribution towards plant pressing and storage in a herbarium is appreciated. *Dr. James Acai* made an important contribution in the peer reviewing of the draft proposal and editing the paper on baseline survey. *Dr. Parick Vudriko* and *Dr. Mathias Afayoa* for their contributions to *invitro* studies and technical audit of the experimental set-up and also, immensely appreciated for quality assurance during the experimental set-up. *Mr. Nathan L. Musisi* is thanked for his contribution to the efficacy studies of microbial activities of the plant extracts on common bacteria. *Ayoo Betty Laura* participated in plants material collection from the four districts in the south western agro-ecological zone of Uganda. *Dr. Nsubuga Mutaka Robert* played crucial roles in the editing and peer review of proposals, baseline studies and criteria to be followed while collecting medicinal plants for laboratory studies.

Mr. Francis Omujal, Mr. Moses Agwaya, Mr. Tumusiime, and *Mr. Corn Amai* are appreciated for their contributions in the plant extraction process and phyto-chemical analysis of the plant extracts. *Dr. Nannyingi O. Mark* his contribution to peer review has been useful in shaping structural adjustments in the paper presentation. *Dr. Sarah Nalule* made useful contributions to efficacy studies and acute toxicity profiles including peer review of the papers.

Her contributions in critiquing philosophical flow and paper patterns have been paramount.

Mr. Kitui James and *Ms. Kibui Pauline* participated in experimental trials and record keeping of all experimental results.

NARO-Mbarara ZARDI management is thanked for hosting the early stages of the research. The staff of *Uganda National Chemotherapeutic Research Laboratories* for assisting us to undertake extraction and qualitative phytochemical analysis at its premises. *Makerere-COVAB:* The Department of Pharmacology and Therapeutics for hosting some of our studies on *invitro* studies and acute toxicity profiles in the Laboratory.

Late Prof. Gary Wassemer for providing technical and structural guidance while he was a visiting Lecturer at MUST in September, 2009. *Ms. Judith Francis (CTA)* for providing us with resource materials, journal papers and books for references and support for reviewing our papers. *Dr. Preston (LRRD)* and *Dr. Ester Gebrekistos* for publishing the baseline study and getting technical personnel to review the paper. The vital role of *Dr. Rita Payan Carreira* and *Kuria Anthony* of Tropical Biology Association, Nairobi are highly appreciated.

District Veterinary Officers: offering favourable support to the research. Veterinary Officers of Mbarara, Ntungamo, Sheemaand Rakai for collecting and supporting every activity of the research while data was being collected in their respective sub counties.

Dr. Simon Anguma for encouraging and supporting us towards the commencement this research piece of work.

Dr. Tolo casim Umba and *Mr. Morgan Andama* for technical peer review and encouragement while undertaking the research. Dr. Dominic Byarugaba; for technical and professional guidance during the research and identifying issues related to ethical standards, royalties, indigenous knowledge technologies and asset benefit and sharing. *Dr. Grace Kagoro* and *Dr. Julius B. Lejju* thanked for their continued guidance and interest in the research piece of work.

Further still, we thank the vital contributions of *Mr. Max O. V. Irama, Mr. John Kisembo* and *Rose Ainembabazi* for their roles in laboratory work. Furthermore, role of *Ms. Rose Alma Palma Ababiku* and *Professor Claire Card* are appreciated for peer reviewing chapters of the book.

The moral support extended to us by *Mrs. Sarah Tusimiire Lagu, Magdalene Anzoa, Philip Lele, Paula Asianzo* and *Pius Opi Manzi* is greatly appreciated.

Last, but not least, appreciation is further extended to *David Amanya, Musa Bright, Twesigye John, Alex Tibenderano* and *Severino Tusiime* who assisted in data collection. *Farmers* and *extension workers from Mbarara, Ntungamo, Sheema* and *Rakai* for being supportive and availing plant materials and information on the use of these plant medicinal extracts.

About the Authors

Charles Lagu
(BVM, MSc. LDPM (MAK), DPAM (UMI), Ph.D.)

Department of Biology, Faculty of Science
Mbarara University of Science and Technology (MUST)
P.O. Box 1410
Mbarara Uganda
Corresponding author: chlaguu@gmail.com

Professor Frederick I. B. Kayanja
(BSc, B. Vet. Med, MSc, Ph.D., DSc (hc) LCP, FRVMA, MRCVS, FAAS, FTWAS, FUNAS)
Department of Anatomy
Faculty of Medicine
Mbarara University of Science and Technology (MUST)
P.O. Box 1410
Mbarara Uganda

List of Tables

LIST OF FIGURES

LIST OF ABBREVIATIONS AND ACRONYMS

%	Percentage
µg	Microgram
µl	Microlitre
^0C	Degree Centigrade
ANOVA	Analysis of variance
BVM	Bachelor of Veterinary Medicine
CBC	Complete blood Count
cm	Centimeters
COVAB	College of Veterinary Medicine Animal Resources and Biosecurity
CTA	Technical Centre for Agricultural and Rural Cooperation
DFID	The Department for International Development
DHP	Dry land Husbandry Project
DMSO	Dimethylesulfoxide
Dr.	Doctor
Ed	Editor
epg	Egg per gram
FAO	Food and Agricultural Organization
FGD	Focus Group Discussion
g	Gram
GDP	Gross Domestic Product
GIT	Gastro Intestinal Tract
HIT	Haemagglutination Inhibition Test
HPI	Heifer Project International
IIRR	International Institute of Rural Reconstruction
ITDG	Intermediate Technology Development Group

ITK	Indigenous Technical Knowledge
KI	Key Informant
l	Litres
LD_{50}	Lethal Dose (50%)
LDPM	Livestock Development Planning and Management
LRRD	Livestock Research for Rural Development
MAAIF	Ministry of Agriculture Animal Industry and Fisheries
MbaZARDI	Mbarara Zonal Agricultural Research and Development Institute
MCHC	Mean Corpuscular Haemoglobin Concentration
MCV	Mean Corpuscular Volume
MHA	Mueller Hinton Agar
MHC	Mean Haemoglobin Concentration
MIC	Minimum Inhibitory Concentration
ml	Milliliter
mm	Millimeter
M Sc.	Master of Science
MUST	Mbarara University of Science and Technology
MVM	Modern Veterinary Medicine
NAADS	National Agricultural Advisory Services
Nacl	Sodium Chloride
NALIRRI	National Livestock Research and Resources Institute
NARO	National Agricultural Research Organization
NCD	Newcastle Disease
OECD	The Organization for Economic Cooperation Development
RBC	Red Blood Cells
Rf	Retardation factor
SPSS	Statistical Package for Social Scientists
SWAEZ	South Western Agro-ecological Zone
TLC	Thin Layer Chromatography
TNF	Tumour Necrosis Factor
t-test	Student t test
TVM	Traditional Veterinary Medicine
UBOS	Uganda Bureau of Statistics
UMI	Uganda Management Institute
UNCRL	Uganda National Chemotherapeutics Research Laboratories
UNHC	Uganda National Housing and Census
UPE	Universal Primary Education

VO	Veterinary Officer
VV	Viscerotropic Velogenic virus
WAAVP	World Association for Advancement of Veterinary Parasitology
WBC	White Blood Cells
ZARDI	Zonal Agricultural Research and Development Institute

ABSTRACT

A lot of medicinal plants are used in poultry disease management. However, information on zone wide medicinal profiles, efficacy, safety, dosage, active substances and effectiveness of these plants are unknown. The study aims to evaluate the effectiveness of two commonly used medicinal plant extracts i.e., *Capsicum annum* and *Erythrina abyssinica* in the control of Newcastle disease and Helminthosis respectively in indigenous chickens in the south western agro ecological zone (SWAEZ) of Uganda.

The Research on *E. abyssinica* indicated that the lethal dose (LD_{50}) of its ethanolic extracts was 3039.23 mg/kg. The clinical signs depended on the level of concentration of the plant extracts. The study concluded that 70% ethanol extracts of *Erythrina abyssinica* were safe to use and were classified as practically nontoxic (5-15g/kg body weight).

Additionally, phytochemical ingredients in *E. abyssinica* root bark, stem bark and leaf and *C. annum* seeds from Mbarara district were analysed and the following bioactive compounds were found present in many of the plant parts viz; tannins; reducing compounds; polyuronides saponins; alkaloid salts; alkaloids; quaternary bases; steroid glycosides; coumarin derivatives; anthracenocides; flavanosides; anthocyanosides. These bioactive chemicals have significant uses in management of poultry diseases.

C. annum was a very useful herbal medicine that could be used to control outbreak of Newcastle disease. Its use is very significant if birds are treated before they are attacked by Newcastle disease virus. *Use* must follow right concentration, dose and standards in mixing the extracts. The extracts should be prophylacticaly administered before the outbreak of the NCD. Alcohol extracts were found to be better than aqueous extracts.

There was up to 60% mortality by NCD in the infected and untreated affected group. Prophylactic treatment with *C. annum* at least one to two weeks before infection mitigates mortality as result of NCD by over 90%. The conventional approaches to vaccinate the birds using thermo-labile and thermo-stable NCD vaccines still work. This method is more effective among the large scale poultry producers. The clinical signs i.e., gross lesions, histopathology, serology all indicated presence of NCD in the infected and untreated group. It was clear that *C. annum* extracts within the safety dosage were not toxic to the liver and kidneys.

E. abyssinica was efficacious in the control of *Ascaridia galli*. It was also effective in the control of *Trychostrongylus tenuis* and coccidian parasites. Generally, haematological and biochemical tests revealed very minimum disturbances in the liver and kidney functions. It can therefore be concluded that, it is safe to use *E. abyssinica* leaf extracts in the control of *A. galli* infections, *Trychostrongylus tenuis* and coccidian parasites. Cases of reinfection for the case of coccidia were very common phenomena. The efficacy of *E. abyssinica leaves extract* were comparable to the conventional drug *Piperazine citrate*. The relationship between the treatment groups and egg per gram reduction was expressed in correlation rank coefficient (r^2), *Erythrina abyssinica* leaves extracts (95.09%), *Piperazine citrate* (92.56%) and negative control (95.43%).

The research recommended appropriate simple, user friendly standardization of the extracts for farmers to apply. Further understanding of the specific bioactive compounds responsible for activity against the parasites is vital. There is need to undertake sub acute and chronic toxicity study on key organs by the plants.

Chapter 1

INTRODUCTION TO POULTRY ETHNOVETERINARY MEDICINE IN UGANDA

ABSTRACT

This chapter introduces the poultry ethnoveterinary medicine. Alternative medicine which is cost effective, and easily accessible in addressing disease burden in poultry, provides insight into the wider field of this part of emerging veterinary field. It further explains the research problems identified as a result of using the conventional approach in the control of Newcastle disease (NCD) and helminthosis. It highlights the objectives of the study, justification, conceptual frame work and scope of the study.This chapter offers an attempt to narrow the information gap that exists between researchers, technicians and family poultry farmers.

1.1. INTRODUCTION

Understanding rural poultry production systems through thinking and innovation is very important in promoting the enterprise. This should aim at getting solutions to poultry farming problems (Tadelle and Ogle, 2001). Poultry makes an important contribution to the livelihood of billions of people world-wide (Kitalyi, 1998; Acamovic et al., 2005; Gueye, 2009). In Uganda, Poultry constitutes a major livelihood source of household incomes and food security (MAAIF, 2000; UBOS, 2006).

Currently, the contribution of agriculture to national gross domestic product (GDP) is 23.7% of which livestock contributes 8% of the national GDP (Uganda Bureau of Statistics, 2009). Livestock products play a key role in raising incomes of households and providing a source of protein to many families. Poultry products recorded an upward trend in production (Uganda Bureau of Statistics, 2009). The national chicken flock for Uganda was estimated to be 37.4 million as of 2008. The western region has 7.2 million chickens (19.3%) of the national flock. The agricultural module of the Uganda National Housing and Census (UNHS) 2005/2006 recorded an estimated chicken count of 23.5 million compared to 37.4 million recorded in 2008. This represents an increase of 13.9 million (37.2%) chickens over this period (MAAIF & UBOS, 2008).

The national ducks flock for Uganda was estimated to be 1.5 million as of 2008. Regionally, western Uganda had 300,610 ducks, 20.6% of the national ducks flock. The national turkey population for Uganda was estimated to be 0.35 million as of 2008. Regionally, western Uganda had the least numbers of turkeys estimated to be 22,000 (6.3%) (MAAIF & UBOS, 2008).

The total chicken numbers by districts in SWAEZ of Uganda include; Rakai (503,623); Sheema (364,568); Mbarara (239,470); Isingiro (203,564); Sembabule (194,462); Ntungamo (184,760); Ibanda (144,301); Kiruhura (142,459); and Lyatonde (73,588) (MAAIF & UBOS, 2008).

Poultry is a micro livestock with the capacity of being multiplied quickly to meet the demands of the population in addition to supplying vital protein requirements in the diet of household communities (Kekeocha, 1984; National Council, 1991; Tadelle & Ogle, 2001; Ramdas, 2009). Poultry eggs have an excellent nutritive value. They contain 12-14% well balanced protein and essential amino acids and contain 10-12% fats with a high percentage of unsaturated fatty acids. Poultry eggs contain 1% minerals mainly iron, phosphorus, calcium and sulphur. Eggs are a good source of Vitamin D, B and about 250 mg of cholesterol (Acamovic et al., 2005).

Poultry is very good start up enterprise. It has a short generation interval and is less expensive to buy than other livestock and livestock products. It has less financial risk and faster return on investment. As a product it has reduced spoilage, efficient use of space, affordable facilities, ease of management and increased productivity (Alders and Spradbrow, 2001; Acamovic et al., 2005; Kolawole et al., 2007; Ramdas, 2009). Poultry enterprises fit well into existing farming systems thereby expanding the resource base and recycling nutrients. Many authorities recommend poultry as one of the enterprises suitable for vulnerable groups (FAO, 2001; NAADS, 2003; Haslwimmer, 2004; Lagu et al., 2011).

Although indigenous chicken play a very significant role in the rural economy, indigenous breeds are known to have poor productivity. A number of factors are responsible for poor productivity and mortalities such as diseases e.g. Newcastle disease (NCD), helminthosis, fowl typhoid etc. Other constraints include predation by wild cats, wild birds and wild dogs. Additionally, lack of feed attributed to the high cost of feed, and failure to provide feeds also contribute to poor productivity. Poor housing attributed to lack of resources to construct housing units. Diseases and parasitism are due to coccidiosis, helminthosis, mites, lice as stated by (Ramdas, 2009). Newcastle disease is responsible for 50-80% annual death of rural flock in many parts of Africa (Kitalyi, 1996; Alders & Pym, 2009; Jordan & Alderson, 2009).

Currently, thermo-labile and thermo-stable New castle vaccines are used for management of the disease (For example, Illango, 2000; Olivier, 2004; Ramdas, 2009). However, these vaccines face poor cold chain maintenance,Also costs involved in catching and vaccinating widely spaced small flocks among the households are high (Kitalyi, 1996; Alders & PYM, 2009). The above problems make the use and application of these vaccines uneconomical.

Other than NCD, helminthosis is another problem affecting productivity of poultry (Alders & Spradbrow, 2001). Helminthosis retards the normal growth rates of indigenous chicks. Helminths consume nutrients of the birds and suck blood from the birds leading to anaemia.

It has been observed that the use of commercial NCD vaccine for control of NCD and the use of commercial dewormers for controlling heminthosis are minimal especially among the typical backyard indigenous poultry farmers.

The typical backyard poultry farmers rely on medicinal plants in the control of NCD and helminthosis (Olila, et al., 2007; Kolawole, et al., 2007). The efficacy and effectiveness of these plant derived medicinal extracts are not well known and therefore not properly documented.

The purpose of the study was therefore to evaluate the efficacy and effectiveness of *E. abyssinica* and *C. annum* commonly used plant derived medicinal extracts for the management of NCD and helminthosis in the south western agro-ecological zone (SWAEZ) of Uganda.

1.2. Statement of the Problem

Despite the fact that control of NCD and helminthosis in indigenous poultry can be managed by use of NCD vaccines and dewormers respectively, these have largely not been effective and sustainable and therefore little success recorded. To make matters worse, these vaccines are not accessible to many poultry farmers especially in rural areas. They are not cost effective to small farmers too, because they are packaged in large doses for 500-1000 birds, a figure out of reach for many small holder farmers who keep 5-25 birds. Relatedly, there was another problem of catching and vaccinating widely spaced small flocks among the households in the villages by the veterinary personnel. The availability of the thermo-stable vaccine to the farmers is still an illusion. Efforts to combat helminths among the indigenous chickens in Uganda faced similar problems. Most smallholder poultry farmers in the south western agro-ecological zone heavily rely on the use of medicinal plants in the control of Newcastle disease and helminthosis. Much as these plant extracts are widely used, little is known about their variety and effectiveness in the control of NCD and helminthosis. The active chemical substances and doses are not known. This makes it very hard for indigenous technical knowledge (ITK) to be widely applied and promoted. The study aimed at the evaluation of the effectiveness of *C. annum* and *E. abyssinica* respectively in the control of New castle disease and helminthosis in poultry in the SWAEZ of Uganda.

1.3. Main Objective of the Study

The study aimed at the evaluation of the effectiveness of *C. annum* and *E. abyssinica* respectively in the control of NCD disease and helminthosis in poultry in the SWAEZ of Uganda.

1.3.1. Objectives

The objectives of the study were:

1. To profile common medicinal plant species used by local farmers in the control of NCD and helminthosis in poultry in the south western agro-ecological zone.
2. To determine the acute toxicity levels of *C. annum* and *E. abyssinica* in the control of Newcastle disease and helminths affecting poultry in the SWAEZ.
3. To identify bioactive compounds in *C. annum* and *E. abyssinica* used in the control of Newcastle disease and helminths affecting poultry in the SWAEZ.
4. To evaluate the effectiveness of *C. annum* and *E. abyssinica* used in the control of Newcastle disease and helminths respectively in the SWAEZ.

1.4. Research Questions

1. What are the common plant species used by local farmers in the control of NCD and helminthosis in poultry in the SWAEZ?
2. What are the optimum concentration levels and toxicity levels of the medicinal plant extracts?
3. What are the phyto-chemical levels of these medicinal plant extracts?
4. How effective are these two plant extracts commonly used in the control of Newcastle Disease and helminths respectively in the SWAEZ?

1.5. Justification

The innovative aspect of indigenous technical knowledge (ITK) is development of appropriate community-based technology for controlling NCD and internal parasites in poultry using indigenous knowledge systems and locally available natural resources. Through conducting clinical (field) trials, this project scientifically established the efficacy of these medicinal plants for management of NCD and helminths. The improvement indicators included reduced mortality rates, increased chick growth rates through cost effective treatment of chicks with utilization of indigenous technologies and local available feed resources. Increased egg production per hen and increased chicken turn over. This was expected to increase the number of farmers engaged in organic poultry production, increase egg and poultry meat output from the system leading to improved household food security, nutrition, incomes and improved welfare of the rural household and contribution of poultry to the national economy and thus poverty eradication.

It was noted that few poultry farmers have direct contact with researchers and technicians and there are few researchers dealing with issues related to family poultry value chain compared with the number of family poultry farmers. This research attempts to narrow the distance between researchers, technicians and family poultry farmers.

1.6. Conceptual Frame work

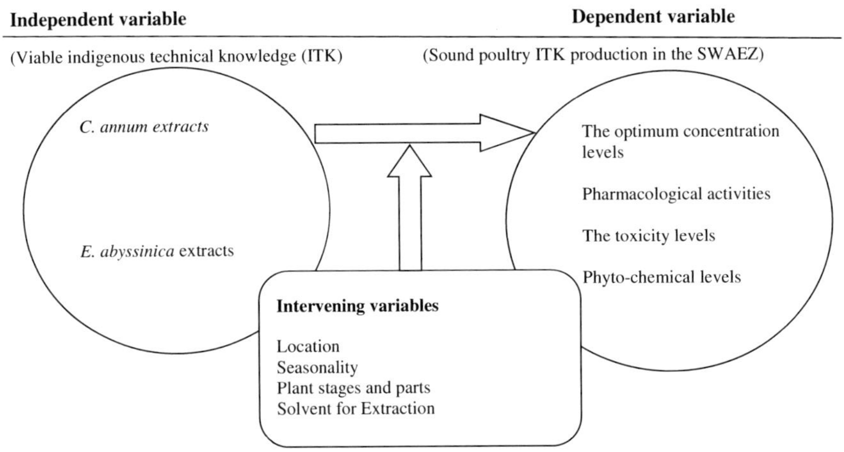

1.7. Scope

This research covered areas related to understanding the phyto-chemical levels, pharmacological activities, the optimum concentration levels and the toxicity levels of extracts of aqueous and ethanolic *C. annum* and *E. abyssinica* extracts. This study provided essential information required in integrating indigenous knowledge in the poultry farming system in the SWAEZ of Uganda. It involved poultry farmers in the districts of Rakai, Ntungamo, Sheema and Mbarara. These districts have the high chicken populations as follows; Rakai (503,623); Sheema (364,568); Mbarara

(239,470); compared to Isingiro (203,564); Sembabule (194,462); Ntungamo (184,760); Ibanda (144,301); Kiruhura (142,459); and Lyatonde (73,588). Data was collected over a period of 12 months, analysis and documentation and final write- up over the next twenty four months. This study was undertaken over a period of three years.

Chapter 2

ETHNOVETERINARY POULTRY LITERATURE REVIEW

ABSTRACT

Indigenous technical knowledge (ITK) or local knowledge is vital to ensuring sustainable resource use and balanced development. ITK may appear simple to outsiders, but it has come of age to represent minimal livelihoods for the rural resource-poor people. A major constraint for advocating for community-based use of herbal medicines for treating livestock diseases and conditions is lack of scientific evidence of their efficacy, and lack of standardized procedures for their application. There are information gaps related to analysis of procedures, effectiveness of herbal medicines, and standardization of herbal medicines and their toxicity levels. Extensive research in this area is key to understanding concerns in this whole range of medicinal plants. This chapter reviews attempts made in this field.

2.1. LITERATURE REVIEW

2.1.1. Indigenous Technical Knowledge (ITK)

Indigenous technical knowledge or local knowledge is important to ensure sustainable resource use and balanced development (Adjanohou et al., 1988; Gbile, 1991; Marcus, 1992; Ejobi and Olila 2004; Wanzala et al., 2005; Ejobi et al., 2007; Kolawole et al., 2007). This view was challenged by earlier theorists, who saw traditional knowledge and institutions as obstacles to development (Wanzala et al., 2005; Kolawole et al., 2007).

Indigenous technical knowledge (ITK) may appear simple to foreigners, but it has come of age to represent minimal livelihoods for the rural resource-poor people. 'ITK provides the basis for local level decision-making, which is most apparent in formal and informal community associations and organizations' (Katunguka-Rwakishaya et al., 2004; Olila et al., 2007; Kolawole et al., 2007).

The need to understand farmers' knowledge, offers a platform for referencing and asking technical and scientific questions in research (Kolawole, et al., 2007). 'It also provides the basis for alternative technologies that are not imposed as alien 'packages', which contradict existing, practices' (Wofgang and Sollod 1986; Wong-Leung 1988; Nuwanyakpa et al., 1990; Nuwanyakpa et al., 1995; Satrija et al., 1995; Olila and Bukenya, 2005; Kolawole, et al., 2007).

One of the indigenous technical knowledge is use of traditional medicine. Traditional medicinal use has lasted since pre-historic times. Majority of world's population use primary forms of human and animal medicine (Wanzala et al., 2005). The development of ethnoveterinary medicine had not matched that of human medicine (McCorkle, 1986). Ethnoveterinary medicine remains an important ethnos-cientific resource to be tapped into for the benefits of the poor rural communities.

McCorkle (1986) and Wanzala et al. (2005) observed that traditional herbal remedies that are efficacious e.g., quinine, picrotoxine, curare and rauwolfia serpentine and herbs like *Combretum mucronatum* and *Mitragyna stipulosa*.

There are, however, certain problems faced by the local farmers who use ethno-veterinary approach to treat their animals. These problems include inconvenience involved in the use or preparation of certain remedies; seasonal availability of certain medicinal plants; paucity of treatment against epidemic diseases; existence of harmful practices; difficulty of standardizing herbal remedies (since the concentration of a critical ingredient in a plant often varies from one location to another); and vagueness of local treatment schedules as highlighted by Kolawole et al. (2007).

The poultry farmers lack preventive and control measures to combat disease outbreaks. It is only during the start of an outbreak that birds are treated using ITK. The effectiveness of ITK used in the control of poultry diseases is not known (Tadelle and Oster, 1996). Guèye (2009) documented gaps that exist in family poultry farmers indigenous knowledge system and that the ITK are limited due to lack of scientific verification, expertise and isolation.

Katunguka-Rwakishaya et al., 2004 documented the great variation in dosage rates among individuals though no cases of overdose had been reported in various livestockdisease management. A range of solvents are used to extract active ingredients from the identified plants e.g. water, ethanol or acetone etc. Many farmers use water to extract active ingredients from these plants and yet water is not the best solvent for extraction because it does not extract all active ingredients. McCorkle (1986) and Wanzala et al. (2005) observed that active substances vary according to location, season, plant parts and growth stages. Root and stem barks may have higher concentration of the active compounds compared to the leaves. This needed to be verified scientifically.

Innovative ideas and programmes are required urgently to promote rural poultry production for the improvement of rural households (Tadelle, 1996; Alders and Pym, 2009; Guèye, 2009). There was urgent call for research interventions in this area for cost effective control of Newcastle and helminths in the farming system in the South Western agro-ecological zone (SWAEZ).

Since indigenous technical knowledge (ITK) is essential for sustainable development, policy makers should enact policies that would enhance the integration of modern health supplies and systems with indigenous knowledge. In addition to this, scientific standardization of ethno-veterinary practices will enhance their acceptance across culture and among stakeholders (Olila, et al., 2007).

The optimum production of indigenous poultry can be achieved through addressing managerial and technical areas of production. These include control of NCD, improved feed system, regular provision of water and provision of small scale night enclosures (Tadelle, 1996; Alders and Pym, 2009).

All the selected ITK plants are endemic to the SWAEZ of Uganda. These plants were selected for the *invivo* studies (field trials) on the basis of previous studies (Katunguka-Rwakishaya, et al., 2004). This study evaluated two plants *C. Annum* and *E. abyssinica* derived medicinal extracts commonly used in the control and management of Newcastle diseases and helminthes respectively in the South Western Agroecological Zone of Uganda (SWAEZ).

2.1.2. Efficacy and Effectiveness of Plant Derived Medicinal Extracts

A major constraint to advocate for community-based use of herbal medicines for treating livestock disease and conditions, are lack of scientific evidence of their efficacy and lack of standardized procedures for their application. In Uganda, considerable efforts in the recent past have been made to document medicinal plants traditionally used in livestock healthcare and production systems.

This work has largely been spearheaded by the Faculty of Veterinary Medicine at Makerere University (Ejobi and Olila, 2004; Ejobi et al., 2007).

Some research on documentation of medicinal plants for animal use has been done by the National Livestock Research Institute (NALIRI) in Tororo. In the Teso sub-region, Ejobi and Olila (2004) documented a total of 182 plants traditionally used for treating livestock diseases and conditions. A recent study by Ejobi et al. (2007) reported a total of 24 plants traditionally used by the Bahiima pastoralists in Rakai district for treating livestock diseases. About 20% of plants reported in that study, were traditionally used for controlling gastro-intestinal parasites. Olila et al. (2007) documented plants traditionally used for treating poultry diseases in the central and eastern regions of Uganda.

Invitro screenings of anti-helmintic bioactivity of some medicinal plants have been conducted in the Faculty of Veterinary Medicine at Makerere University (Igga, 2007). The results were quite promising and exciting. Out of the 8 plants screened for anti-helmintic bioactivity (using the *Ascaris suum* test model), 6 showed significant anti-helmintic bioactivity; with worm mortalities ranging from 50 to 100% following a 24-hour exposure period to the crude plant extracts studied. However, clinical/field trials have not been conducted to demonstrate the efficacy of these plant extracts using livestock models. There is therefore no strong scientific evidence for promoting use of these herbal remedies among livestock keeping households.

Elsewhere in the world, literature is rich in herbal remedies developed and promoted for use in livestock healthcare (Satrija et al., 1995; Marcus, 1992; Gbile, 1991; Wong-Leung, 1988; Wofgang and Sollod, 1986). In Cameroon, for example, the Heifer Project International (HPI) initiated an Ethno-veterinary Medicine/Fulani Livestock Project in 1989 to seek sustainable alternatives for animal health and production problems (Nuwanyakpa et al., 1990). That initiative was triggered by, among others, expensive and erratic supply of veterinary drugs and supplies experienced by the HPI (Nuwanyakpa et al., 1995). That project tested, and promoted the utilisation of medicinal plants (*Terminalia schriperiana* and *Vernonia amygdalina*) for control of gastro-intestinal helminths in cattle (Nuwanyakpa et al., 1995).

Katunguka-Rwakishaya et al. (2004) compared albendazole, a commercial anthelmintic and plant anthelminthic extracts. The plant anthelminthic was able to reduce the worm burden by 57-65% of the original egg per gram (epg). This could provide an alternative means of helminths control in reducing worm egg count output.

A study by Mtambo et al. (1999) evaluated a combination of *Capsicum annum* (red pepper), *Citrus limon* (lemon) and *Opuntia vulgaris* (prickly pear) against Newcastle disease (NCD) in domestic fowl. The results indicated that there was no prophylactic or therapeutic value of the plant extract against NCD. The plant extract showed a negative effect on body weights in birds with NCD.

The pharmacological activities of these plants probably boost the immune system and exhibit bactericidal and antihelmintic properties. The effects of the plant extracts on animal resistance to disease or infection may be explained by other activity rather than instant action on the bacteria, virus or worms only. The extracts may enhance the action of useful bacteria so that the overall effect of the burden by the virus or worm is reduced. These ideas need scientific investigation.

2.1.3. Toxicity Levels of Plant Derived Medicinal Extracts

McCorkle (1986) and Wanzala et al. (2005) noted that plant extracts are taken to be safe and the dose is not sometimes regulated. This may lead to toxic and other side effects like diarrhoea. Are these plants always safe even during egg laying periods? And if not at what level should they be recommended to farmers?

There are information gaps related to analysis of procedures, effectiveness of herbal medicines, and standardization of herbal medicines and their toxicity levels. Extensive research in this area is key to understanding concerns in this whole range of medicinal plants Gueye (2002); Ramdas (2009).

Ramdas (2009) noted that prevention of losses due to diseases was a solution to indebtedness among indigenous communities and strengthening local livelihood. The role of multi and interdisplinarity is essential to understand the use of these plants for management of diseases (Guèye, 2009; Ramdas, 2009).

The root bark and leaves of *E. abyssinica* were reported as traditionally being used by some Bahiima cattle keepers in Rakai District in the South Western rangelands for controlling worms in livestock (Ejobi et al., 2007).

Chapter 3

MATERIALS AND METHODS IN POULTRY ETHNOVETERINARY

ABSTRACT

This chapter attempts to explain the Study Design, Study area and how sample size was determined. It adequately describes the medicinal plants, *C. annum* and *E. abyssinica*. It explains how sample collection was done, Preparation of crude plant extract, standardization of dosages, clinical (field) trials and experimental study including the laboratory analysis of fecal and blood samples. The use of *C. annum* to control NCD in birds in the SWAEZ, toxicity of the extracts and compounds, identification of phyto-chemical properties of *C. annum* and *E. abyssinica*, statistical analysis and considered key information and guides in ethical considerations during the research were done.

3.1. STUDY DESIGN

The experimental design employed probability sampling, data collection, analysis and reporting. Households in the sub counties, parishes and villages were selected with the guidance of local extension officers and local leaders. A multistage sampling technique was used to characterise the households that used ITK. A stratified sample of households that used the ITK was selected for the studies that run for at least 12 months. The next 24 months period was for data analysis and reporting.

3.2. Study Area

The research was located in south western rangelands of Uganda covering the districts of Rakai (Luanda; GPS GPS Location 36M 0329859 UTM 9925403, Elevation 1195m); Ntungamo (Rubare; GPS S00^{0}59.007^1 E030^{0}2.230^1, Elevation 1397m); Mbarara (Rubindi S00^{0}18.589^1 E 030^0 35.322^1 Elevation 1396m); and Sheema (Bugongi; S00^{0}36.309^1 E030^{0}36.774^1 Elevation 1395m) that had a high population of indigenous chickens according to the livestock census conducted by UBOS and MAAIF (2008).

3.3. Sample Size Determination

A total of 400 day old chicks were bought and kept semi intensively till they attained 4 months. The birds were fed and also allowed to scavenge for the rest of the day while growing like those birds kept under the traditional indigenous poultry rearing system. After 4 months the grown up birds were randomly selected in representative samples for the randomized experimental trials.

3.4. Description of the Medicinal Plants

3.4.1. Capsicum annum L (Solanaceae)

Common Name: pepper

Runyakole name: Eshenda, Madi Names: Kiyita. *Capsicum annum* is a perennial shrub which grows to 2 m (6') with a woody trunk. Leaves have various shapes but are usually elliptical up to 10 cm (4") long. Flowers are white to yellowish in groups of 2 or 3 and followed by small, upright, fiery, green fruits that ripen to red. The varieties of the "fruit" vary greatly in size, color and pungency.

The plant is propagated through the seed. The part of the plant that provides therapeutic action is the seed oil. The active ingredient in the plant is *capsaicin* that is used for the management of medical conditions.

3.4.2. *Erythrina abyssinica* Lam.ex DC (Leguminosae)

Described by Augustin Pyramus de Candolle in 1825. *Erythrina abyssinica* (Runyakole name: *Ekiko*), is a deciduous savannah species in the family of leguminosae. It grows in open woodland and grassland. It has characteristic red overflowing flowers. It can be propagated through seedlings, cuttings and truncheons. In the SWAEZ of Uganda, it is sometimes planted along fences of paddocks to support barbed wires. It has various traditional medicinal applications in livestock. It is also used in traditional human medicine. The bark of young stems is used to treat trachoma. It is also roasted and applied to burns and swellings. Powdered root is used for syphilis, anthrax, and snakebites.

3.5. Sample Collection

Fresh samples of the plant materials to be studied were collected from the fields. The samples included seeds and leaves of *Capsicum annum* and root bark, stembark, leaves, of *Erythrina abyssinica*. During field collection of the samples, the sites where the plants were found were geographically and ecologically described. Ejobi et al. (2007) found that these plants were abundantly found in all areas in the South Western rangelands. The plant *Erythrina abyssinica* and *Capsicum annum* were identified and verified by a Botanist from Mbarara University of Science and Technology. The collected samples were stored at the Botany herbarium unit.

The quantity of each plant biomass to be collected approximately corresponded (per dosage) with the amount of plant biomass traditionally used in the current traditional practice. The plant materials were kept in a plant press, and then transported to the Pharmacology Laboratory of the Faculty of Veterinary Medicine, Makerere University for the extraction procedures. Voucher specimens of the plants studied were deposited in the laboratory with Voucher numbers as described in 5.2.2.

3.6. Preparation of Crude Plant Extract

The crude extracts were prepared as follows: The fresh plant material was dried on top of laboratory benches for about 7 days. The material was ground using a laboratory grinder (Model: Brook Crompton series 2000, UK) to yield a fine free flowing powder. The powder was weighed, and soaked in a known volume of 70% ethanol.

The samples were allowed to stand for about 4 days while being gently shaken in an automatic shaker This was followed by filtering using Watman® filter paper No. 1. The solvent was removed using a rotary evaporator (Buchi-RE-111, Switzerland) and under reduced pressure. The crude extracts were weighed, and percent yield of the crude extract calculated as:

$$\text{Percent yield} = \frac{\text{Weight (g) of Crude extract X 100}}{\text{Weight of plant material extracted}}$$

This crude extract was used for the experimentation (clinical/field trials) with the identified chicken in the management of NCD and helminthosis in the SWAEZ.

3.7. Standardization of Dosages

The data on the percent yield of the crude extracts were used for standardizing dosage rates of fine powder preparations of the plant materials. For example, the amount of crude extract contained in a known weight of fine powder of plant material was calculated.

3.8. Clinical (Field) Trials

The indigenous chickens were allowed to acquire the parasites viz; *Ascaridia galli, Strongylus species, coccidial infections* naturally from the areas where they scavenged.

Their parasite load before administration of experimental treatment was ascertained by fecal examination using the McMaster technique. This elucidated the effect of varied parasite intensity and spectrum as it occurred under farmers' husbandry practices.

3.9. Experimental Study

A completely randomized design was used for the clinical trials as described by Thrusfield (2003). Before experimentation (natural infestation), the study indigenous chicken worm load levels were established by fecal sample analysis using the Mc Master technique.

Worm infested chicken were allocated to three experimental groups, using age and weight as blocking factors. Group 1 (n=35) was assigned to treatment with the crude plant extracts, and administered as a single oral dose, group 2 (n=35) was the positive control and was treated with *piperazine citrate* and the third group (n=35) was the negative control. The experimental chickens were identified using numbered collars. Weights of the chicken and fecal eggs per gram (e.p.g.) were determined.

During the experimental phase (each lasting a total of 28 days), the study chicken were housed in individual pens, and intensively fed. The chicken had acclimatized to the pens before the beginning of the experiments. The fecal and blood samples were collected on days 0 (before treatment), 7, 14, 15, 21 and 28. The study chickens were weighed each week for 6 consecutive weeks.

The fecal samples or droppings were collected from the cloaca, and preserved in 10% formalin until analyzed.

At the end of the experimental period, one chicken from each experimental group was sacrificed, and a detailed post-mortem examination carried out. Content of the gastro-intestinal tract recovered were taken for detailed examination of the spectrum of helminths present. Dose scaling of the crude extract were performed before the experimental study as described by Lagu and Kayanja (2013b).

3.10. Laboratory Analysis of Fecal and Blood Samples

The fecal samples were analyzed in the Mbarara Medical Specialists Laboratory. The worm loads were determined using the MacMaster slide. The roots were harvested for crude extraction using ethanol (70%). The crude extracts were used in the poultry for testing and evaluating for efficacy. The worm load determination was done at day 0,7,14, 15, 21 and 28 intervals. Relatedly blood samples for total blood cell count and biochemical analysis were undertaken at the College of Veterinary Medicine, Animal Resources and

Biosecurity (COVAB), Makerere University (MAK) and results compared among the treatment groups.

3.11. The Use of *Capsicum annum* to Control Newcastle Disease in Birds in the SWAEZ

The trials were conducted at Mbaguta cell, Ruharo Ward, Kamukuzi Division, Mbarara Municipality. An experiment was set up to test the *Capsicum annum* on selected and identified reared free range chicken placed under five treatment groups. Blood samples in two tubes with non coagulant and anticoagulant were collected from the birds under five treatment groups on days 0, 4, 7, 10, 14, 18, 21. NCD titer baseline and subsequent titers established from blood samples as per allocated days. The collected blood samples were taken for laboratory analysis at the COVAB, Makerere University in a cold chain. Results of titre values, total blood cell count and biochemical analysis of the sampled blood were compared among the different treatment groups.

3.12. Toxicity of the Extracts and Compounds

To determine the toxicity of the extracts, 25 mice were used as experimental animals. The mice were kept in a separate unit at room temperature i.e., 25 ^{0}C with a 12 hours light and dark cycle for 4 weeks to acclimatize. The rats had access to food and water *ad libitum.* The freeze dried extract was administered orally using tubing attached to a syringe. Varying dosage rates of the plant extracts were given. Observations were made on food intake or consumption patterns, general behaviour and any gross pathological toxic effects on internal organs.

Pathologic effects were recorded. Blood collected and liver function tests assessed to detect variation in key indicator enzymes. At the end of 15 days, the mice were sacrificed and major organs like the heart, liver, kidney, brain and muscles collected for histo-pathological examination. Lethal doses LD_{50} were computed as a dose at which 50% of the test animals would die.

3.13. Extraction of Phyto-Chemical Properties of *Capsicum annum* and *Erythrina abyssinica*

Solvents of polarities (Houghton and Raman, 1998) to extract a diversity of compounds from the plants were selected. The polar solvents used were technical grade ethanol, acetone, methanol and water; three apolar solvents used were dichloro methane, hexane and phenyl ether. For the initial screening process, 10 g sample (leaf, stembark or root were extracted with 50 ml of the respective solvent while vigorously shaking on an orbital shaker for 1 hour.

Aqueous extraction of the dry ground plant material in distilled water was done for about 1 hour. The un-extracted material was separated by centrifugation. Filtration was done to obtain a filtrate and the supernatant extract pre-weighted in glass bottles. The organic solvents evaporated in a stream of air at room temperature over night to determine the mass extracted. Water extracts were dried in a vacuum drier. The weight of the extracted material was always measured.

3.14. Characterization of the Active Compounds in *Capsicum annum* and *Erythrina abyssinica*

Dried extracts were re-dissolved in the corresponding solvent to yield a 10 mg/ml solution. An aliquot of 10μl of each solution (i.e., 100 μg) was applied on thin a layer of chromatography (TLC) plates. Compound separation was effected by solvent eluent systems. On the TLC plates, separated compounds were inspected and marked under visible and ultraviolet light.

During preparative TLC, the plate was subsequently sprayed by suitable spray reagents (vanillin, methanol and concentrated sulphuric acid), and thereafter heated in an oven at 100^0C for few minutes to optimal colour development. Data on content was grouped as root, stembark and leaves to assess if any differences in concentration existed. Silica gel was used for column chromatography. To assess the biochemical content variation sample analysis was done using materials collected.

3.15. Statistical Analysis

The data on faecal eggs per gram (epg) counts were entered into Microsoft Excel. The data were subjected to general linear (repeated measures) model analyses using SPSS. Independent T-test at 5% level of significance was used to test for differences in the treatments and time periods. Descriptive statistics was computed. Similar statistical analyses were performed to test the differences in weight gains in the experimental treatment groups.

Data on the titre values, mortality rates and weights were collected and entered in SPSS version.11 and Genstat and analyzed for descriptive statistics and inferential statistics (frequencies, cross tabulations, chi-square, correlations, regressions, ANOVA and t-test). This was used to draw conclusions on their effectiveness as far as controlling NCD and helminthosis was concerned.

3.16. Ethical Considerations

The research was approved by the ethical Science committee of Mbarara University of Science and Technology. The committee also approved the use of specimen animals for the research.

Additionally, the recommendation of World Association for the Advancement of Veterinary Parasitology (WAAVP) was used in conducting efficacy and toxicity studies. The intellectual property rights policy of MUST was adhered to. There was respect and adherence to data and information generated from poultry farmers who participated in the survey study. The data was stored carefully and confidentially. The data generated were used only for purposes of the study.

Chapter 4

Acute Toxicity Assessment of Ethanolic and Water Extracts of Leaves of *Erythrina abyssinica* (Leguminosae) in the South Western Agro-Ecological Zone of Uganda

Abstract

This chapter indicated that the lethal dose (LD_{50}) of ethanolic extracts of *E. abyssinica* was 3039.23 mg/kg. The clinical signs noted depended on the level of concentration of the plant extracts. The study concluded that 70% ethanol extracts of *E. abyssinica* were safe to use and were classified as practically nontoxic (5-15 g/kg body weight). The extracts were suitable for poultry disease management by farmers. Further toxicity studies using chicken as animal species were necessary. Sub-acute and chronic toxicity tests were recommended in order to determine the long-term effects of the extract. The 70% ethanolic extracts of *E. abyssinica* had a lethal dose (LD50) of 3039.23mg/kg.

4.1. Introduction

Many in-vitro studies indicated that many medicinal plants are efficacious (Wasswa & Olila, 2006; Lagu and Kayanja, 2010). *E. abyssinica* has wide spread use as herbal concoctions by small holder farmers. Many of the formulated concoctions are unstandardised and hence have wide dose ranges.

A wide range of medicinal plant users do not appreciate the fact that their extract can be toxic to the body. Standard laboratory tests by Joshi et al. (2007) indicated profound toxicity in some plant extracts.

The study hypothesized that medicinal plant with unknown toxicity levels exist in the SWAEZ of Uganda. The study therefore aims to assess the acute toxicity levels of *Erythrina abyssinica* in the SWAEZ. The establishment of toxicity levels of *E. abyssinica* is crucial to ascertain the safety of the *E. abyssinica* extracts.

4.2. Materials and Methods

4.2.1. Data Collection

The leaves of *E. abyssinica* were collected from Mbarara district. The collected materials were pressed and voucher specimen deposited at the Botany Department at Mbarara University of Science and Technology. The rest was taken taken to Mbarara Zonal Agricultural Research and Development Institute (MbaZARDI) for drying. The plants were dried under the shade for one week at room temperature of about 25^0C. The plant materials were then pounded into powder (in a mortar) for chemical extraction at the Uganda Natural Chemotherapeutics Research Laboratories (UNCRL).

4.2.2. Plants Identification and Experimental Setup

The *E. abyssinica* were collected and identified by a botanist. The extraction was conducted using ethanol. The extracts were administered under various doses to mice. The experimental set up included positive and negative controls. The ethical committee of Mbarara University of Science and Technology approved the use of experimental animals for the test experiment.

4.2.3. Extraction of Active Ingredients and Determination of Extraction Efficiency

250 g of the freshly dried powdered leaves of *E. abyssinica* were macerated in 2000 ml of 70% ethanol for 72 hours with intermittent shaking.

Filtration through cotton wool was done to remove coarse particles (residues) followed by filter paper 12.5 mm (Whitman®, No.1). The filtrate was concentrated on Rotary evaporator (Buchi-RE-111, Switzerland) under reduced pressure at 40^0C. The concentrated extracts were later dried on weighed kidney dishes to a constant weight at 50^0C. The above procedures were repeated with water as the solvent. The dried extracts were packed into universal bottles and kept at 4^0C until needed for bioassays. Acute toxicity effects *of E. abyssinica* were investigated in the Division of Pharmacology and Physiological Sciences, COVAB, Makerere University.

4.2.4. Acute Toxicity Study Protocol

Swiss albino mice of 16-25 gr body weight of both sexes were selected and labelled using markers of different colours on the tail. The animals (n=30) were divided into six groups of six mice each and kept in different cages for easy observation. The dose levels were determined after a preliminary acute toxicity trial, which had been carried out earlier. The doses rates were as shown below (9.2.5).

4.2.5. Preliminary Acute Toxicity Levels of Crude Extracts of *Erythrina Abyssinica*

Treatment groups	Dose levels (mg/kg)	n	No. dead
Group 1	2000	6	
Group 2	4000	6	
Group 3	6000	6	
Group 4	8000	6	
Group 5	10,000	6	
Control	1 ml dH2O	6	

The volumes of the drug doses administered to the mice were calculated using the following formula (Ghosh, 1984): Volume (mls) = body weight (kg) x dose levels (mg/kg)/stock drug concentration (mg/ml).

The derived dose levels for ethanolic extracts were 2,000, 4000, 6000, 8,000, 10,000 mg/kg.

4.2.6. Data Collection and Analysis

Mortality (number of dead mice) were counted in each group and recorded. The median lethal dose that killed 50% of the test animals was determined using the graphical and probit analysis. Any signs of toxicity observed in the collected organs were also recorded.

4.2.7. Postmortem Procedure

The numbers of dead mice after being subjected to the medicinal plants crude extracts (*E. abyssinica*) under varying dose level concetrations were noted. Randomly selected animals (n=2) from each group were submitted to necropsy for organ collection. The surviving mice were sacrificed and subjected to post mortem analysis. Within 24hrs, organs from mice that died or were sacrificed were collected and fixed in jars containing formalin (10% formaldehyde) and subsequently submitted to routine paraffin-embedding. Organs collected for histopathology were liver, kidney, lungs, intestines and brain.

Four (4) micrometer sections of the collected organs were routinely stained with haematoxylin and eosin for histological examination, performed by a Pathologist. Putative histopathological changes in the structural organization of the liver, kidney, lungs, intestines and brain were observed and recorded.

4.2.8. Histo-Pathological Analysis

Samples of liver, kidney, lungs, intestines and brain were fixed in 10% neutral formalin and processed by conventional techniques. Paraffin sections (6 μ) were stained with haematoxylin and eosin before microscopic examination.

4.2.9. Quality Assurance

The calyces were shade dried to prevent loss of essential chemical components and the voucher specimen were taken to the herbarium (Biology Department, Mbarara University of Science and Technology) for identification and also to ensure quality techniques adopted from World Health Organization (WHO) guidelines on herbal quality control. The ethanolic extracts of *E. abyssinica* leaves were kept in sterilized bottles and placed in a refrigerator at 4°C to prevent mould formation. All the reagents used were analytical grade.

The swiss albino mice of the same age were used for the study to minimize variation in the test results. The control group given 1 ml of distilled water was used for comparison with the groups given the plant extract.

4.3. Results Presentation

4.3.1. Signs recorded during acute toxicity studies were: increased motor activity, anaesthesia, tremors, arching and rolling, clonic convulsions, ptosis, tonic extension, lacrimation, Straub reaction, exophthalmos, pilo-erection, salivation, muscle spasm, opisthotonus, writhing, hyperesthesia, loss of righting reflex, depression, ataxia, stimulation, sedation, hypnosis, cyanosis and analgesia.

Collection of Organs for Histopathology

The postmortem study was done within 24 hrs on dead animals and those that survived. Organs for histopathology were fixed in 10% formalin. These included liver, kidney, lungs, intestines and brain. The Lethal dose (LD_{50}) was calculated according to Fisher's and Yates (1948) as illustrated in Table 1.

Table 1. Results on the acute toxicity of *Erythrina abyssinica*

Acute Toxicity assessment of *Erythrina abyssinica*					
Percentage yield for Leaves 2.85%					
Group	Extract solution (mls)	No. Dead out of 6	% Dead	Log dose	Probit
1	2,000	0	0	3.3	3.3
2	4,000	1	33.33	3.6	4.56
3	6,000	3	50	3.78	5
4	8,000	4	66.67	3.9	5.42
5	10,000	6	100	4	7.33

GRAPH FOR LD_{50} DOSE

y=mx + c............................Equation v Substituting in the equation,

y= 0.1738 (3.78)+2.8258

y= 3.482764

Antilog y= 3039.23 mg/kg

According to y-axis y=5 in which our calculated x value=3.482764 in which the ld_{50} is its antilog.

Ld_{50} is equal to the antilog 3.482764 of which is approximately 3039.23 mg/kg

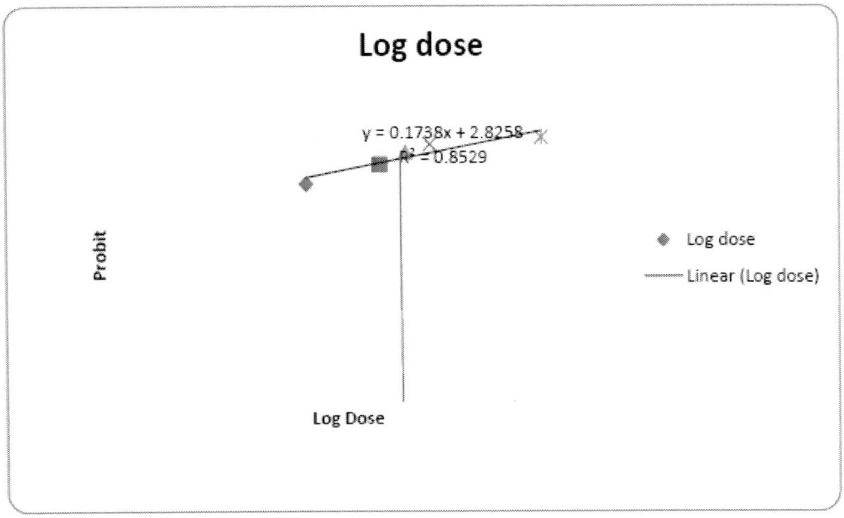

The lethal dose was established to be 3039.23 mg/kg
Ld_{50}=3039.23 mg/kg

4.3.2. Histopathological findings of *Erythrina abbysinica* leave extracts

Organ	Normal organ	Key significant pathological findings
Brain	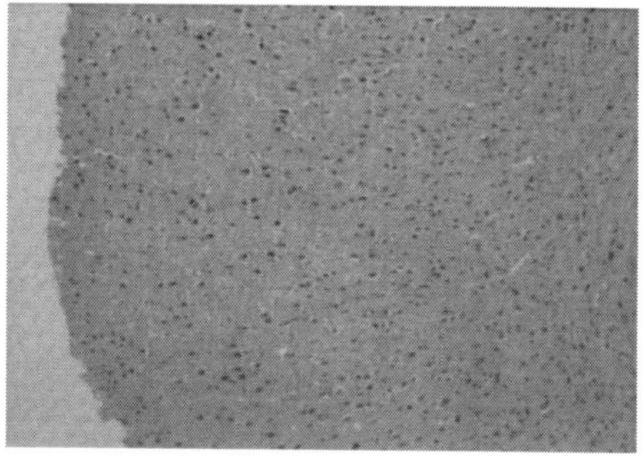 Negative control Brain (Cerebrum). The Scale bar is 100 µm	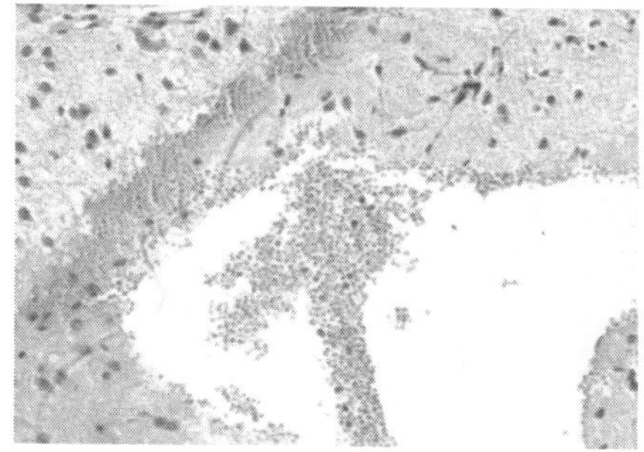 Hemorrhages in the Cerebrum .The Scale bar is 100 µm
Intestines	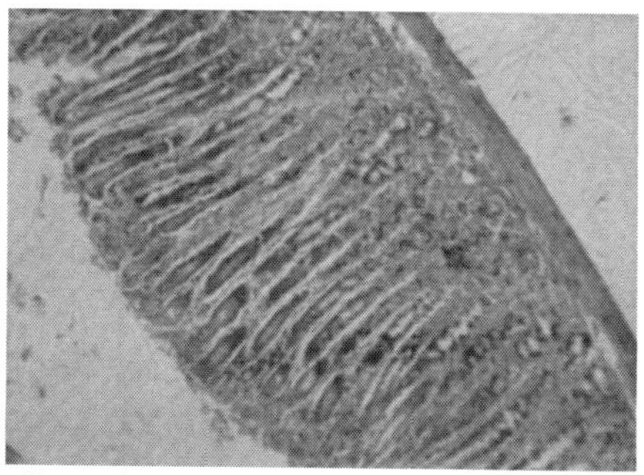 Negative Control (Intestines).The Scale bar is 100 µm	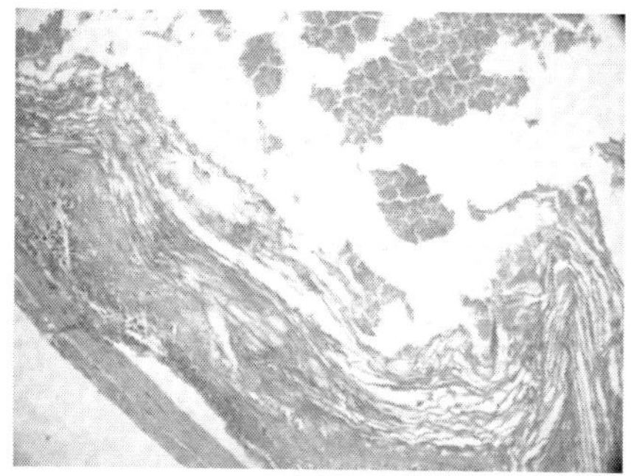 Severe hemorrhages on the intestines.The Scale bar is 100 µm

Organ	Normal organ	Key significant pathological findings
Kidneys cortex	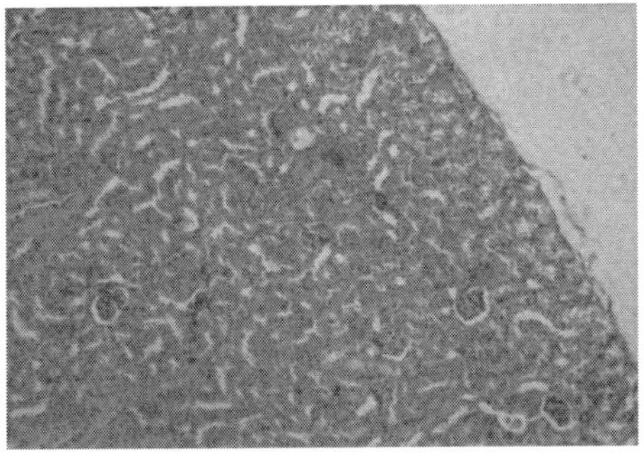 Negative control Kidney cortex.The Scale bar is 100 μm	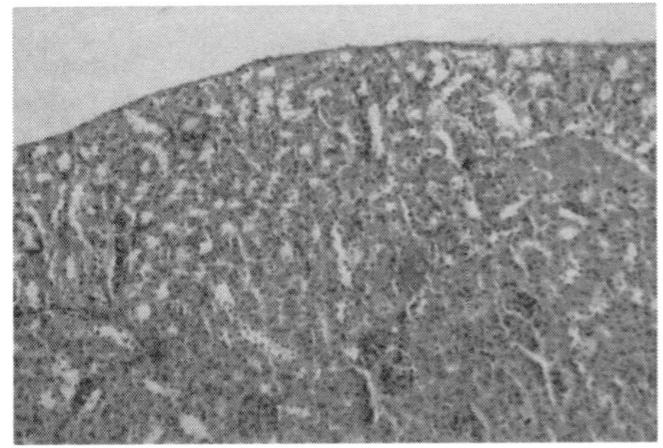 Haemorrhages and congestion in the Kidney cortex.The Scale bar is 100 μm
Kidney medulla	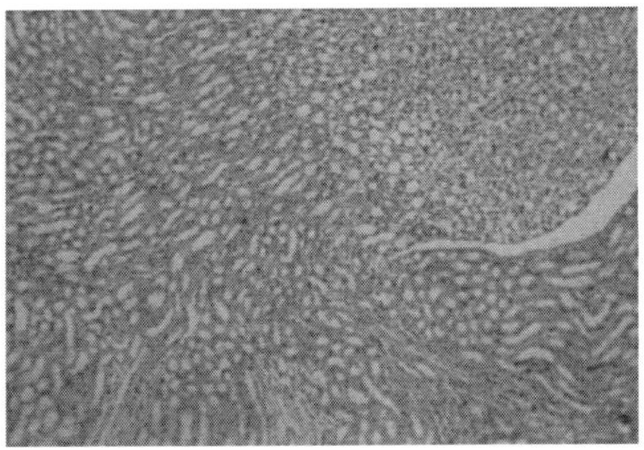 Negative control kidney .The Scale bar is 100 μm	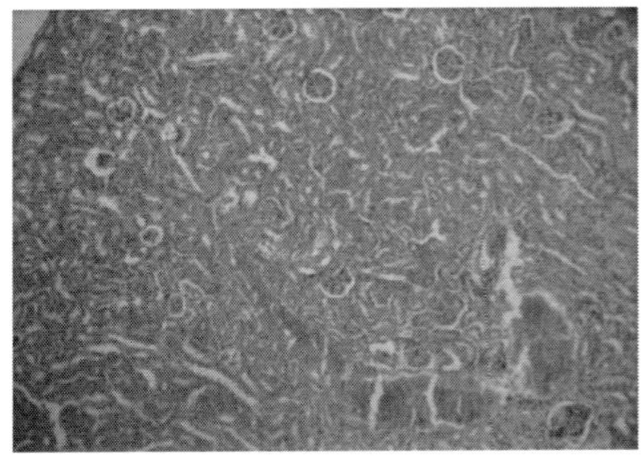 Hemorrhages, congestion in the Kidney medulla.The Scale bar is 100 μm

Organ	Normal organ	Key significant pathological findings
Liver	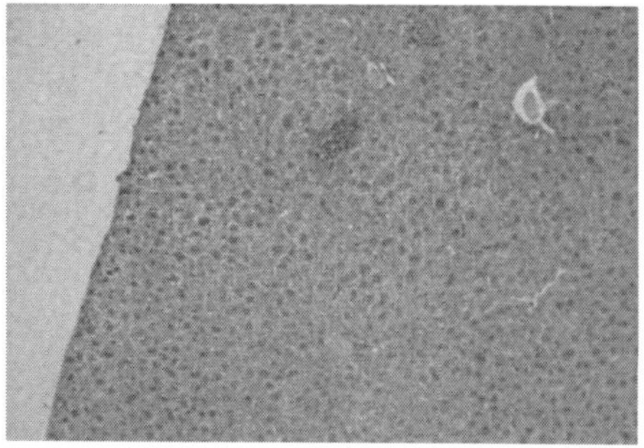 Negative control (Normal liver).The Scale bar is 100 μm	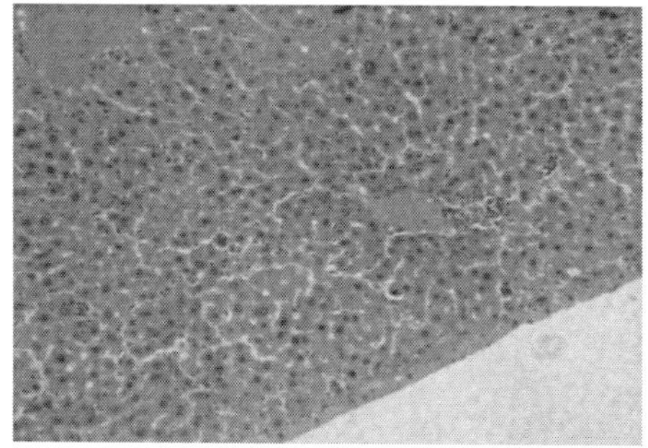 Multifocal areas of Liver necrosis and degeneration.The Scale bar is 100 μm
Lungs	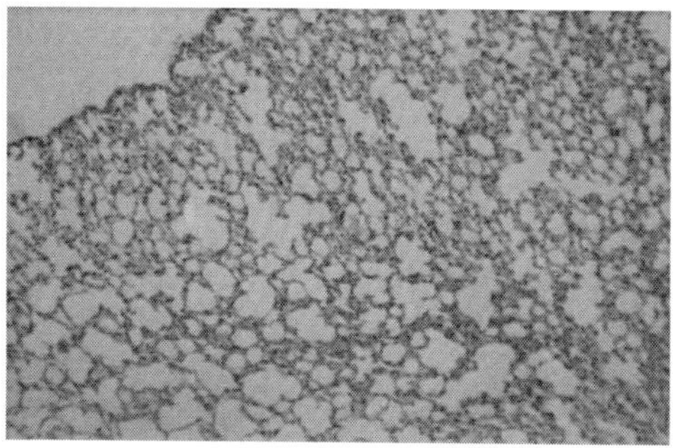 Negative control lungs.The Scale bar is 100 μm	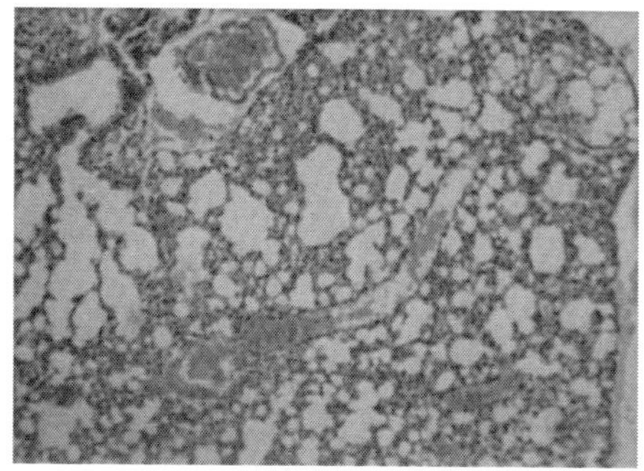 Lung congestion and hemorrhages.The Scale bar is 100 μm

RESULTS DISCUSSION

4.4. LETHAL DOSE (LD_{50}) LEVELS

The 70% ethanolic extracts of *E. abyssinica* had a lethal dose (LD_{50}) of 3039.23 mg/kg. According to Gosh (1984), *E. abyssinica* is classified as practically non toxic because the LD50 results lie in the dose range of 5-15 g/kg body weight.

Local small holder farmers are using ethanolic extracts of *E. abyssinica* seeds to manage various ailments. This study has validated that the use of the ethanolic leaves extract of *Erythrina abyssinica* by the communities is safe. It is to be noted that the dose levels greatly vary from one farmer to another as does the method of extraction (Lagu and Kayanja, 2012). The farmers' dose levels are much lower than the determined LD50 of 3039.23 mg/Kg body weight for ethanolic extracts.

The Organization for Economic Cooperation Development (OECD) Guidelines for the Testing of Chemicals (1995), recommends that the maximum dose level for any chemical compounds should not exceed 5000 mg/ Kg body weight of an animal. The ethanolic extraction of *E. abyssinica* has advantages compared to water use because ethanol is a better extraction solvent for bioactive compounds which is in agreement with the findings of Harbone (1984); Bizimenyera et al. (2007); Bussmann et al. (2011) and Chandra et al. (2010).

After administration of high extract doses often there were notable clinical signs in the test animals. Key clinical signs noted were irritation shown by the use of fore limbs to scratch the areas of the mouth, gasping for air, dyspnoea, twitching of GIT muscle, urination, dry mouth, reddening of lips and convulsions. The effect of bioavailability of the drugs on major organs like the intestines, liver, lungs, kidneys and brain were a clear manifestation of the presence of active substances in these major organs.

The histopathological findings showed significant effects on the brain, kidney, lungs, small intestines, liver and heart. Results by Joshua et al. (2010) in India indicated that necropsy examination are paramount in linking the general and target organ specific toxic effects of phytomedicine. Many others are in agreement (OECD, 2000; Gad, 2007; Hayes, 2007 and Monjanel-Mouterde et al. (2006)).

CONCLUSION

Results of the study indicated that the lethal dose (LD_{50}) of ethanolic extracts of *E. abyssinica* was 3039.23 mg/kg. The clinical signs noted were responses by the mice to increased concentration of the plant extracts in the body tissues of the mice. The pathological signs observed in those mice which died could be due to intense accumulation and concentration of the bioactive compounds in the organs well above the safety margin. The surviving mice had none to mild pathological sign of toxicity. The study concludes that 70% ethanol extracts of *E. abyssinica* are safe to use and are classified as practically nontoxic (5-15 g/kg body weight). Extracts are suitable for poultry disease management by farmers. Further toxicity studies using chicken as animal species is necessary. Sub-acute and chronic toxicity tests are recommended in order to determine the long-term effects of the extract.

Chapter 5

PHYTO-CHEMICAL ANALYSIS OF PLANT EXTRACTS OF *ERYTHRINA ABYSSINICA* AND *CAPSICUM ANNUM* IN THE SOUTH WESTERN AGRO-ECOLOGICAL ZONE OF UGANDA

ABSTRACT

This chapter highlights the phytochemical ingredients in *E. abyssinica* root bark, stem bark and leaves and *C. annum* seeds from the SWAEZ. The plant parts were collected from Mbarara district. The plant parts collected were dried, analysed and the following bioactive compounds were found present in many of the plant parts viz; tannins; reducing compounds; polyuronides saponins; alkaloid salts; alkaloids; quartenary bases; steroid glycosides; coumarin derivatives; anthracenocides; flavanosides and anthocyanosides. These bioactive chemicals were found to have numerous uses in management of livestock diseases especially NCD and helminthosis. There was need to study in detail the role of the pharmacological actions of the individual ingredients in each plant part.

5.1. BACKGROUND

The importance of medicinal plants as sources of new drugs has always been recognized (Soetan and Aiyelaagbe (2009). The problem of drug resistance is rampant both in humans and animals. The use of medicinal plants for management of various human and animal ailments cannot be disputed as observed by (UNESCO, 1996); Schmincke (2003). Natural biodiversity resources in most African countries are rich in medicinal plants. It is observed that 25% of the drugs in modern pharmacopeia are of plant origin (Okigbo et al., 2008).

Synthetic analogues are often developed on prototype compounds that are isolated from medicinal plants. The potential toxicity of medicinal plants or herbs has not been keenly considered by farmers or other medicinal plant practitioners (O'Hara et al., 1998). It is necessary to study the presence of bioactive compounds of the root bark, stem bark and leaves of the plant *E. abyssinica* and seeds of *C. annum*.

Phyto-chemical studies of the plant preparations are paramount for standardization. They aid knowledge on importance of phyto-constituents in reference to observed activitity (Mojab et al., 2003). Phyto-chemistry further helps in standardizing the herbal preparations so as to get the optimal concentrations of known active bio-constituents and complex chemical substances (Birdi et al., 2006; Soetan and Aiyelaagbe, 2009). It helps widen horizons in the value of ethno medicinal remedies in livestock disease control.

Standardization can be done by obtaining a chemical fingerprint/profile. Chemical fingerprints through chromatographic techniques are more commonly used for standardization and are obtained in terms of one or more marker compound (Birdi et al., 2006; Banso and Adeyemo, 2007); Soetan and Aiyelaagbe, 2009). The study determined the bioactive chemical constituents of *E. abyssinica* and *C. annum*. The study hypothesized that some medicinal plants in the SWAEZ have different bioactive compounds varying with plant parts and species.

5.2. Materials and Methods

5.2.1. Sample Collection, Preparation and Extraction

The samples of *E. abyssinica* leaf (2 kg), *E. abyssinica* stembark (2 kg) and *E. abyssinica* root bark (2 kg) and *C. annum* seed (1 kg) were collected from Mbarara district. The samples were dried under shade for 14 days. The dry samples were then reduced to powder using an electric grinding machine (Model: Brook Crompton series 2000, UK) before extraction. The samples were extracted by maceration of *E. abyssinica* leaf (100 g), *E. abyssinica* stembark (100 g) and *E. abyssinica* root bark (100 g) and *C. annum* seed (100 g) in 500 ml of 70% ethanol for 72 hours at room temperature. The solution was filtered with whatman filter paper No.1. The product was then concentrated to half volume and tested for different phytochemicals.

5.2.2. Phytochemical Analysis

Using ethanol extracts, two sets of analysis were performed. One set involved analysis in fresh ethanol extract while the other involved analysis in 70% ethanol extracts following the method by (Harbone, 1984).

5.2.3. Analysis on Ethanol Extract

Test for tannins

Ethanol extract (1 ml) was diluted with water (4 ml). Ferric chloride (3 drops) was then added. The occurrence of a blackish blue color or green blackish color indicated the presence of tannins (Harborne, 1984).

Test for Reducing Compounds

Ethanol extract (1 ml) was diluted with water (2 ml). Fehling's solutions I (1 ml) was added followed by Fehling's solution II (1ml). The product was heated in a water bath at 90°C. Formation of a brick-red precipitate denoted the presence of reducing compounds in the sample (Harborne, 1984).

Test for Polyuronides

Ten ml of ethanol extract was added, drop wise, to water (5 ml) and shaken to allow formation of a thick precipitate. The precipitate was separated by filtration using whatman filter paper and washed further with water. The residue precipitate obtained on the filter paper was stained with hematoxylin. Formation of a violet or blue color was an indication of presence of polyronides or mucilages (Harborne, 1984).

Test for Saponins

Ethanol extract (2 ml) was placed in a test tube and diluted with water (2 ml). The product was shaken for about 15 minutes. Formation of a foam (soap like) column of about 2 cm above the liquid level in the test tube indicated the presence of saponins (Harborne, 1984).

Test for Alkaloid Salts

Ethanol extract (15 ml) was dissolved in 10% v/v Hydrochloric acid (10 ml).The alkaloids from the sample were precipitated from the aqueous solution as bases with the help of 10% v/v ammonia solution (10 ml). The solution was extracted with diethyl ether (15 ml) by shaking in a separating funnel. The ether solution fraction was evaporated to dryness in a water bath. 2% hydrochloric acid solution (3 ml) was added to the dry test tube to dissolve the alkaloids. The acidic solution was then divided into three position of 1ml and 2-3 drops of Mayer's reagents was added to one portion. Formation of opalescence or a yellowish-white precipitate in test portion compared to other portions confirmed the presence of alkaloid salts (Harborne, 1984).

Test for Alkaloids & Quartenary Bases

Ethanol extract (10 ml) was mixed with 10% hydrochloric acid (10 ml). The solution was refluxed for about 15 minutes and allowed to cool. Sodium chloride (5 g) was added to the solution, stirred and filtered with filter paper (Harborne, 1984).

Test for Alkaloids*:* The acidic solution was transferred to the separating funnel and 10% ammonia solution –pH 8-9 (10 ml) added. The solution was then shaken with diethyl ether (10 ml) and allowed to separate. The ether extract was evaporated to dryness in a water bath. 1.5 ml of 2 HCl was added and divided into three portions of 0.5 ml. To one portion 2 drops of Mayer's reagent were added and presence of yellow or whitish grey precipitate indicated presence of alkaloids (Harborne, 1984).

Test for Quartenary Bases*:* The alkaline solution was acidified with 10% HCl (15 ml) and filtered using whatman filter paper. The solution was then extracted with diethyl ether (10 ml) in a separating funnel. The diethyl ether extract was evaporated to dryness and cooled. 2% HCl (1.5 ml) was added to dissolve the residue which was divided into three portions of 0.5 ml each. To one of the portions Mayer's reagent was added and formation of a yellow to whitish precipitate indicated presence of quartenary bases (Harborne, 1984).

5.2.4. Analysis on Hydrolysed Ethanol Extract

Hydrolysis Procedure

Ethanol extract (25 ml) was mixed with 10% v/v hydrochloric acid (15 ml) and refluxed for 30 minutes. The refluxed solution was cooled and extracted with diethyl ether (36 ml) in portions of 12 ml each. The ether extract was dehydrated using anhydrous sodium sulphate (10 g). The dehydrated ether extract was used to test for presence of anthracenosides, coumarin derivatives, steroid glycosides, and flavanoside phytochemicals (Harborne, 1984).

Test for Anthracenosides

The ether extract (4 ml) was concentrated to 2 ml in water and shaken vigorously with 25% v/v ammonia solution (2 ml). The solution was allowed to stand for about 5 minutes. Formation of a cherry-red solution in the bottom layer indicated the presence of emodols (aglycones of anthracenosides) in an oxidized form (Harborne, 1984).

Test for Coumarin Derivatives

Ether extracts (5 ml) was evaporated to dryness in a water bath. Distilled water (4 ml) was added the product heated in the water bath. The solution was cooled and divided into two portions. To one portion in a test tube 10% v/v ammonium solution (2 ml) was added. The occurrence of a blue or green fluorescence under UV light deeper for the alkaline test solution indicated the presence of coumarin derivatives in the sample (Harborne, 1984).

Test for Steroid Glycosides

Ether extract (10 ml) was put in a dry test tube and evaporated to dryness in a water bath and allowed to cool. Acetic anhydride (1 ml) and chloroform (1 ml) were then added to the dry test tube and allowed to stand for 15 minutes. Concentrated sulphuric acid (2 ml) was added by means of a pipette to the bottom of the tube (Liebermann – Buchard's reaction). Formation of a reddish-brown or violet-brown ring at the contact zone of the two layers and a green or violet supernant layer indicated the presence of steroid glycosides (Harborne, 1984).

Test for Flavonosides (Flavone glycosides)

An Ether extract (5 ml) was evaporated to dryness in a water bath. 50% methanol (4 ml) was added to the test tube and heated for about 2 minutes and allowed to cool. The solution was divided into two portions. To one portion metallic magnesium ribbon (0.5 g) was added followed by 5 drops of concentrated hydrochloric acid. Formation of a red or orange solution in the test portion indicated presence of flavonols or flavanones (Shibata's reaction) (Harborne, 1984).

5.2.5. Thin Layer Chromatography (TLC)

Preparation of the Plates

Thin layer chromatography plates were prepared using silica gel. The plates were prepared manually by spreading slurry of silica gel on clean glass plates using a thin layer chromatography machine. The thickness of the plate was 0.25 mm. The coated plates were allowed to dry at room temperature. The dry TLC coated plates were then heated in the oven for 45 minutes to activate the silica gel and remove all moisture. The plates were allowed to cool before being used for spotting the samples for finger printing.

Spotting of Samples on the TLC Plate

A straight line was marked at 2 cm from the bottom of the TLC plates using a pencil. This line was used as a spotting line. Another line was marked 10 cm from the first one and this line indicated the end of TLC solvent front. The solvent front is the distance moved by solvent system on the TLC plate. The samples were then spotted on the bottom line of TLC plates separated by 1cm using standard capillary tubes. After spotting the samples, the plates were dried using an UV lamp for about 5 minutes before planting in the TLC chamber.

5.2.6. Running the TLC System in Chamber

The solvent system to run the TLC plate was selected as chloroform - methanol (50:50), acetone- methanol - chloroform (10:25:5), xylene - diethyl ether (50:50), xylene-diethyl ether-chloroform (15:15:5). The TLC chamber was first washed with soap and dried in the oven and allowed to cool. The solvent system was mixed and put in the TLC chamber, covered and allowed to saturate for 30 minutes before putting in the spotted plates with the samples. After saturating the TLC chamber with solvent system, the spotted plates were dipped carefully into the solvent system and allowed to stand straight in the TLC chamber. The system was then covered and allowed to run for about 30-40 minutes depending on the solvent system. Once the solvent front had reached the solvent second plate mark, the running TLC plate was removed for detection of the spots.

Detection of the plates

The spots were detected using normal visible day room light and UV lamp. After detecting the spots' retardation factor (Rf) values were measured (Harborne, 1984).

$$Rf = \frac{\text{Distance moved by spot}}{\text{Solvent front}} \times 100$$

5.3. RESULTS

5.3.1. Phytochemical Ingredients in *Erythrina Abyssinica* Root Bark, Stem Bark, Leaf and *Capsicum Annum* Seeds

The phytochemical ingredients in the samples of *Erythrina abyssinica* rootbark stembark and *leaf* and that of *Capsicum annum* seeds from Mbarara district are presented in Table 2.

Table 2. Phytochemical ingredients in *Erythrina abyssinica* root bark stem bark and *leaf* and *Capsicum annum* seeds from Mbarara district

Phytochemical bioactive ingredient	*E. abyssinica* root bark	*E. abyssinica* stem bark	*E. abyssinica* leaf	*Capsicum annum* seed
Tannins	(++)	(+)	(+)	(-)
Reducing compounds	(++)	(++)	(++)	(++)
Polyuronides	(+)	(-)	(-)	(-)
Saponin	(-)	(-)	(++)	(++)
Alkaloid salt	(++)	(+)	(++)	(++)
Alkaloids	(+)	(+)	(+)	(+)
Quartenary bases	(-)	(++)	(++)	(++)
Steroid glycosides	(++)	(++)	(-)	(++)
Coumarin derivatives	(++)	(++)	(++)	(++)
Anthracenocide	(++)	(++)	(-)	(+)
Flavanosides	(++)	(+)	(++)	(++)
Anthocyanosides	(++)	(+)	(++)	(+)

Note: (++) Strong positive, (+) Positive, (-) not detected.

5.3.2. TLC Finger Printing *E. Abyssinica* Leaf 70% Ethanol Extract

Table 3(a). Solvent systems: xylene-diethyl ether (50:50); Solvent front: 5.6 cm

Spot	Rf value	Visible light	UV lamp
1	0.82	Orange	Red
2	0.80	Green	Fluorescence blue
3	0.71	Yellow	Red
4	0.25	-	Fluorescence blue

Table 3(b). Solvent chloroform-methanol (50:50); Solvent front: 5.0 cm

Spot	Rf value	Visible light	UV lamp
1	0.97	Green	Red
2	0.83	Orange	Grey
3	0.41	Green	Grey

Table 3 (c). Acetone - chloroform-methanol (10:5: 25); Solvent front: 6.0 cm

Spot	Rf value	Visible light	UV lamp
1	0.82	Light green	Red
2	0.25	Light green	Fluorescence blue
3	0.17	Light green	Fluorescence blue

Table 3(d). Xylene – diethyl ether – chloroform (15:15: 5); Solvent front: 4.0 cm

Spot	Rf value	Visible light	UV lamp
1	0.86	Green	Red
2	0.81	Colorless	Fluorescence blue
3	0.41	Green	Red
4	0.05	Green	Fluorescence blue

5.3.3. TLC Finger Printing 70% Ethanol Extract of *E. abyssinica* Root bark

Table 4(a). Solvent system: chloroform-methanol (50:50); Solvent front: 6.0 cm

Spot	Rf value	Visible light	UV lamp
1	0.97	Orange	Fluorescence blue
2	0.85	Orange	Green
3	0.33	Brown	Grey

Table 4(b). Solvent system: xylene-diethyl ether (50:50); Solvent front: 5.0 cm

Spot	Rf value	Visible light	UV lamp
1	0.76	Yellow	Fluorescence blue
2	0.75	Red	Blue
3	0.73	Yellow	Fluorescence blue
4	0.63	Brown	Fluorescence blue
5	0.03	Brown	Fluorescence green

Table 4(c). Solvent system: Acetone - chloroform-methanol (10:5: 25); Solvent front: 6.0 cm

Spot	Rf value	Visible light	UV lamp
1	0.92	Yellow orange	Green
2	0.25	Green	Fluorescence
3	0.17	Green	Fluorescence

Table 4(d). Solvent system: xylene – diethyl ether – chloroform (15:15: 5); Solvent front: 4.0 cm

Spot	Rf value	Visible light	UV lamp
1	0.83	-	Fluorescence blue
2	0.78	Red	Green
3	0.75	Brown	Fluorescence blue
4	0.61	-	Fluorescence blue
5	0.08	Brown	Violet

5.3.4. TLC finger printing of *E.abyssinica* stem bark 70% ethanol extract

Table 5. Solvent system: chloroform-methanol (50:50); Solvent front: 6.0 cm

Spot	Rf value	Visible light	UV lamp
1	0.90	brown	Fluorescence
2	0.82	Orange	brown
3	0.23	Orange	Grey

5.3.5. TLC Finger Printing 70% Ethanol Extract of *Capsicum Annum* Fruit

Table 6(a). Solvent system: chloroform-methanol (50:50); Solvent front: 6.0 cm

Spot	Rf value	Visible light	UV lamp
1	0.98	Orange	Fluorescence
2	0.85	Orange /yellow	Orange
3	0.40	Light brown	Green

Table 6(b). Solvent system: xylene-diethyl ether (50:50); Solvent front: 5.0 cm

Spot	Rf value	Visible light	UV lamp
1	0.76	Red	Red
2	0.73	Red	Fluorescence blue

Table 6(c). Solvent system: Acetone - chloroform-methanol (10:5: 25); Solvent front: 6.0 cm

Spot	Rf value	Visible light	UV lamp
1	0.87	Light green	Fluorescence
2	0.42	Light green	Fluorescence
3	0.25	Light green	Fluorescence

Table 7. Solvent system: xylene – diethyl ether – chloroform (15:15: 5); Solvent front: 4.0 cm

Spot	Rf value	Visible light	UV lamp
1	0.82	Green	Red
2	0.79	Orange	Fluorescence

5.4. DISCUSSION

5.4.1. Phytochemical Ingredients in *Erythrina Abyssinica* Root Bark Stem Bark and Leaves and *C. Annum* Seeds

The results of the phytochemical ingredients in the samples of *E. abyssinica* root bark, stem bark and *leaves* and that of *Capsicum annum* seeds from Mbarara district are presented in Table 2.

The results indicated that the phytochemicals present in *E. abyssinica* root bark, stem bark and leaves and that of *Capsicum annum* seed ethanol extracts were similar except saponins which were not present in *E. abyssinica* root and stem bark ethanol extracts, polyuronides were not present in *E. abyssinica* stem bark and leaf ethanol extract, steroid glycosides and anthracenosides which were not present in *E. abyssinica* leaf extract and quartenary bases not present in root bark extract of *E. abssinica* ethanol extract as illustrated in Table 2.

Although most of these phytochemicals were present in samples, some were more abundant than others. For example, there was more abundance of tannins in the root bark of *E. abyssinica* compared to *E. abyssinica* stem bark and leaf. Likewise, there was more abundance of alkaloid salts in *E. abyssinica* root bark, *E. abyssinica* leaf and *Caspsicum annum* compared to *E. abyssinica* stem bark.

Tannins are produced to a greater degree by all plants. The harsh, astringent taste of tannin laden bark and leaves makes them unpalatable to insects. Tannins contract the tissues of the body. They draw the tissues together and improve their resistance to infection (Harbone, 1984; Meng et al., 2009; Athanasiadou et al., 2001). Coumarins are powerful smooth muscle relaxants. Anthraquinones have an irritant laxative effect on the large intestine, causing contractions of the intestinal walls and stimulating bowel movements. Flavonoids are anti-inflammatory and are especially useful in maintaining healthy circulation and strenthening capillary walls (Harbone, 1984; Mojab et al., 2003; Meng et al., 2009). This explains the medicinal uses of these extracts.

Saponins are of two types i.e., triterpenoid and steroidal saponins. They have marked hormonal activity and triterpenoid saponins are often strong expectorants, and may also aid in the absorption of nutrients. Cardiac glycosides such as digitoxin, digoxin and gitoxin have a strong direct action on the heart, helping to support its strength and rate of contraction when it is failing. Cardiac glycosides are also significant diurectics. They help transfer fluids from tissues and the circulation to the urinary system (Harbone, 1984; Mojab et al., 2003; Meng et al., 2009).

Steroid glycosides are helpful sedatives and have relaxant effect on the heart and muscles in small doses. They contribute to the ability to suppress and soothe irritant coughs. Alkaloids mostly contain a nitrogen-bearing molecule (-NH2) that makes them particularly pharmacologically active. Some are well known drugs and have a recognized medical use. Some alkaloids are used to treat cancer and others have direct effect on the body, reducing spasms, relieving pain and drying up bodily secretions (Harbone, 1984, Meng et al., 2009).

The TLC finger prints for *E. abyssinica* leaf, stem and roots at 70% ethanol extract are illustrated in (Tables 3a-5). The TLC finger prints for 70% ethanol extract of Capsicum annum fruit are detailed in (Tables 6a-7).

Conclusion and Recommendations

Phytochemical ingredients in *E. abyssinica* root bark, stem bark and leaves, and *Capsicum annum* seeds from Mbarara district were analyzed and the bioactive compounds were found present in many of the plant parts viz; tannins; reducing compounds; polyuronides saponins; alkaloid salts; alkaloids; quartenary bases; steroid glycosides; coumarin derivatives; anthracenocides; flavanosides; anthocyanosides. These bioactive chemicals are known to have various uses in management of livestock and human diseases. There is need to study in details the role of the pharmacological actions of the individual ingredients in each plant part.

Chapter 6

IN VIVO EFFICACY OF CRUDE EXTRACTS OF *CAPSICUM ANNUM* IN INDIGENOUS CHICKEN INFECTED WITH NEWCASTLE DISEASE VIRUS

ABSTRACT

Capsicum annum seed extracts are very useful herbal medicine to control outbreak of Newcastle disease. The use of *Capsicum annum* is very significant if birds are treated before they are attacked by Newcastle disease virus. The use of *C. annum* must follow the right concentration, dose and standards in mixing the extracts. The extracts should be pre administered (prophylactic treatment) before the outbreak of the NCD. Alcohol extracts performed better than aqueous extracts.

In groups, especially the infected and untreated, there was up to 60% mortality in the affected groups. For the infected groups, it was clear that NCD was a big problem affecting the farmers. Prophylactic treatment with *C. annum* at least one week post infection reduces mortality by over 90%.

The conventional approaches to vaccinate the birds using thermo-labile and thermo-stable vaccines still work. The clinical signs, gross lesions, histopathology, serology all indicated presence of NCD in the infected and treated group. It was clear that *C. annum* extracts were not toxic to the liver and kidneys. The study revealed that with increasing time post viral inoculation in the test birds, the antibody titres correspondingly increased drastically hence offering solid immunity. The study recommended farmer friendly packages developed to guide farmers in the administration of the herbal *C. annum* concoctions and their popularization.

6.1. Introduction

Free range indigenous poultry plays an important socio-economic role in 80% of the developing countries like Uganda (Petrus et al., 2011). The demand for indigenous poultry meat and eggs is on the increase (Mwakapuja et al., 2012). The productivity of the indigenous poultry is greatly derailed by diseases and other management factors. The low nutritional status and predation add to morbidity and mortality experienced by the small holder farmers (Alfred et al., 2012).

The greatest constraint to indigenous chicken production is Newcastle disease. It decimates up to 80-85% of the total flock per household annualy (Spradbrow, 1993; Gueye, 2002). The control measures used to manage Newcastle disease (NCD) include vaccination, and good husbandry practices. The vaccination includes use of thermo labile and thermo stable Newcastle disease vaccines (Gueye, 2002; Mwakapuja et al., 2012).

In many developing countries like Uganda, the traditional system of chicken rearing is predominant (Gajendran and Karthickeyan, 2009). The traditional system generally faces challenges related to maintaining the cold chain facility for thermo labile vaccines due to lack of electricity (Illango et al., 2008). The thermo stable vaccines, which could solve this problem, are difficult to access (Gueye, 2002; Mwakapuja et al., 2012). The majority of the small holder farmers keep small numbers of indigenous chicken (5-20) per households. This makes it difficult to buy vaccine doses which are to serve 500 or 1000 birds per vaccination schedule. It should also be noted that the majority of the small holder farmers are fragmented. It is difficult for extension workers to organize to undertake vaccination for large groups at a go to absorb the vaccines without wastage.

A number of medicinal plant preparations are commonly used by smallholder farmers to control Newcastle disease (Street et al., 2008; Lagu and Kayanja, 2010). The fruits of *C. annum* have been used against NCD in Tanzania. Aloe species have been extensively used in Kenya to control a number of chicken diseases, Newcastle being one of them (ITDG and IIRR, 1996). A number of rural communities use *C. annum* and *C. frutescens* as crude extracts to control Newcastle disease.

It was however noted that scientific validation of the *invivo* efficacy of the crude extracts of *Capsicum annum* in Uganda and particularly SWAEZ of Uganda has not yet been done. It should also be noted that many of the small holder farmers use unstandardized doses for treating the Newcastle disease. The farmers also use different mixtures including pure *C. annum* pure, plus water, *Capsicum annum* water extract; *C. annum* water extract with ash added; *C. annum* and mixture with aloe species; *C. annum* plus *T. nicotiana* water extract.

The study hypothesized that *Capsicum annum* has both therapeutic and prophylactic effects on Newcastle disease virus. The study aimed to evaluate the efficacy of crude extracts of *Capsicum annum* in indigenous chicken affected by the Newcastle disease.

6.2. Materials and Methods

6.2.1. Rearing of the Experimental Chicken

A total of 400 one day old local chicks were purchased from a local supplier from Kampala and reared at Ruharo ward, Mbarara Municipality (GPS Location S00^{0}35.998^1 E030^{0}37.690^1 Elevation 1448 m). The day old chicks at the time of purchase were not vaccinated against Newcastle disease (NCD). The chicks were placed in a brooder for three weeks. In the brooder they were given optimal environmental conditions and fed on chick mash (chick and duck mash). From four weeks onwards the birds were fed on growers mash.

The chicks after attaining two months were routinely released outside the poultry house to scavenge as under the extensive free range system. On regular basis the birds accessed green plants and insects from the soils. The birds were de-beaked to prevent cases of cannibalism and other vices. They were kept until they attained the age of 16 weeks (4 months) without being vaccinated against NCD. A total of 200 birds were vaccinated using conventional thermolabile NCD vaccine and the remaining 200 birds were not vaccinated against NCD. The vaccinated and unvaccinated birds were kept separately in two different units.

6.2.2. Experimental Design

Two replicate experiments were conducted. In the first experiment 90 local chickens were labelled using plastic wing-tags made of local plastic materials. The birds were weighed and screened for antibodies against NCD using the haemaglutination inhibition test (HI) (Allan and Gough, 1974). The chicken were randomly assorted into five trial groups namely TG1, RG1 (pre-treated and infected), TG2, RG2 (infected and untreated), TG3, RG3 (infected and treated), TG4, RG4 (uninfected and untreated) and TG5, RG5 (Infected and vaccinated with NCD). Groups TG1-TG5 and replicate groups (RG1-RG5) elsewell had 18 chickens per treatment group. The detailed experimental protocol is illustrated in Figure 1.

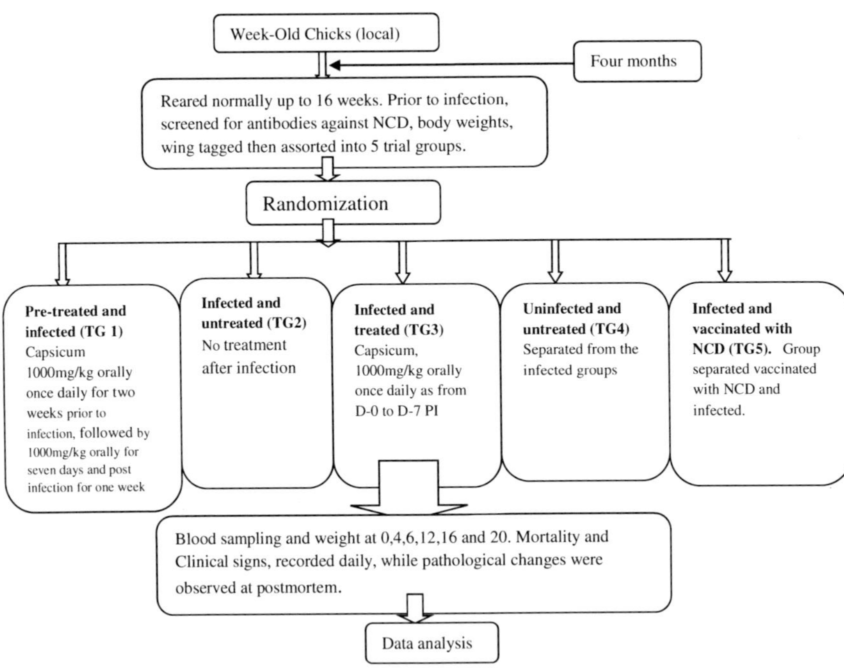

Figure 1. Experimental protocol.

6.2.3. Inoculum for Infection

The local chicken of TG1, TG2,TG3 and TG5 (experiment 1) and RG1, RG2, RG3 and RG5 (experiment 2) were infected with 1ml of 9 log 10 NCD virus containing an effective infective dose of virulent strain $10^{5.6}$. The Pathology Department of the College of Veterinary Medicine, Animal Resources and Biosecurity (COVAB) provided the viral strain that was formerly isolated from local chicken in South Western Agro-ecological Zone (SWAEZ), Uganda and characterized as viscerotropic velogenic (VV) (Yongolo, 1996; Waihenya et al., 2002). The virulence of the viral isolates were tested by first inoculating the virus into embroyonated chicken eggs causing viral multiplication that led to the death of the embryo as described by OIE (1996); Waihenya et al. (2002).

6.2.4. Preparation of *Capsicum annum*

The *Capsicum annum* was obtained from Mbarara District which is located in the SWAEZ. The ripe fruits were collected in a container. A voucher specimen was identified in the herbarium of the Biology Department, Faculty of Science, of Mbarara University of Science and Technology (MUST) and was indexed as Mba Ca001. Approximately 5kg of the ripe fruits of *Capsicum annum* was collected for the experiment. The collected fruits were stored and dried at room temperature i.e., 25°C for one week. The extraction method simulated that which was used in ethno veterinary medicine and also as documented by (Lagu and Kayanja, 2012).

6.2.5. Infection and Treatment Schedule

The same experimental protocol (Figure 1) was used in both experiments. Experiment 2 was carried out to validate the findings from experiment 1.

Parameters Recorded

Following inoculation, clinical signs and mortality rates were monitored daily and postmortem examination was done on dead chicken. Live body weights and blood samples were obtained from chicken on days 0,4,6,12,16 and 20. The serum obtained was investigated for antibodies against Newcastle disease virus using the haemglutination inhibition test (HI) (Allan and Gough, 1974). The standard antigen used in HI was prepared locally at the Pathology and Central Virology Laboratory, COVAB, Makerere University. Most measurements were concentrated on days 0-12 as 80% of the chicken in all groups was expected to have died by day 12. The serum samples were tested and results in addition to replicate results were compared to ensure reliability of the results from the laboratories at COVAB. The wing vein sites were disinfected with iodine solution to prevent contamination and infection. The blood samples were collected from wing veins of the experiemental chicken using a sterile needle both in specimen tubes without anticoagulant and those with coagulant (EDTA). The collected blood samples were kept in a cool box and taken to central labaoratory of COVAB, Makerere University for analysis. For haematological tests using white blood cell counter machine (automatic counter Sysmex, K21. Tokyo, Japan), whole blood in vacutainers with EDTA was used. For biochemical analysis, serum was used to undertake liver and kidney function tests using an automated analytical machine and Liver function test machine (COBAS INTEGRA 400, Germany).

6.3. Data Analysis

Data was entered in Microsft Excel windows 2007. It was exported to Genstat Discovery Edition version 14.1 (Gentat, 2011) where Analysis of Variance was conducted with unbalanced designs. The Cofficient of variation, means, least significance difference at 5% level was analyzed. The summary data of the results were then tabulated. Paired t-test was conducted for comparison of two equal sized sets of data. Graphical analysis and representation of data was done using Micro-soft Excel program. The results of clinical signs and mortality rates, body weights, pathological lesions, antibody levels were summarized and discussed holistically to represent the efficacy of *C. annum* on NCD in the local chicken.

6.4. Results Presentation

6.4.1. Clinical Signs

The observable clinical signs were noted among the two replicates of infected with NCD virus and infected and untreated (TG2 &RG2) with NCD virus and treated groups. Early clinical signs were observed 4 days post infection (PI) whereby up to 40% of the chicken from the two groups appeared weak, drowsy (Figure 2) and showed drooping feathers. There were no observable clinical signs among the pre-treated and infected group (TG1&RG1), infected and vaccinated with NCD (TG5&RG5) and uninfected and untreated (TG14&RG4) in the first 7 days of the start of the experiment. In many of the affected birds from day 5 post infection, there was evidence of dullness, swollen eyelids (Figure 3), anaemia, greenish diarrhea, respiratory rales/ sneezing among the birds that were brought together. In all cases of the birds that showed clinical observable signs of NCD, there were clear signs of greenish diarrhea and torticolis (Figure 4). There was one case of a bird in the infected and vaccinated with NCD vaccine (TG5) that showed weakness, drowsiness, respiratory rales, and coughing, sneezing and swollen eyelids. However, this particular bird in the (TG5) group did not die. In the three groups (TG2, TG3 and TG5) where birds showed clinical signs, the combs and wattles darkened.

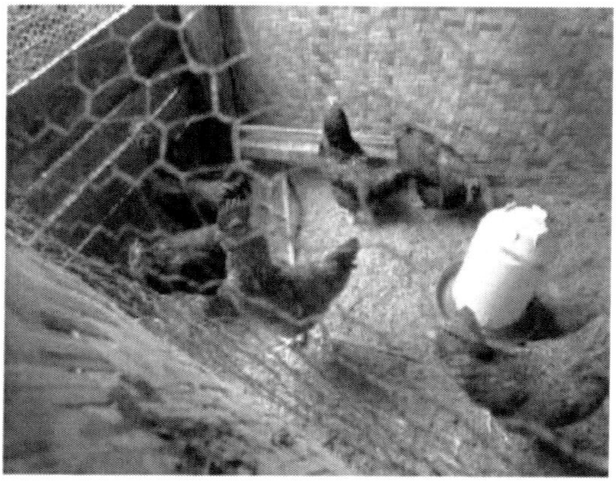

Figure 2. Birds drowsing in the pens.

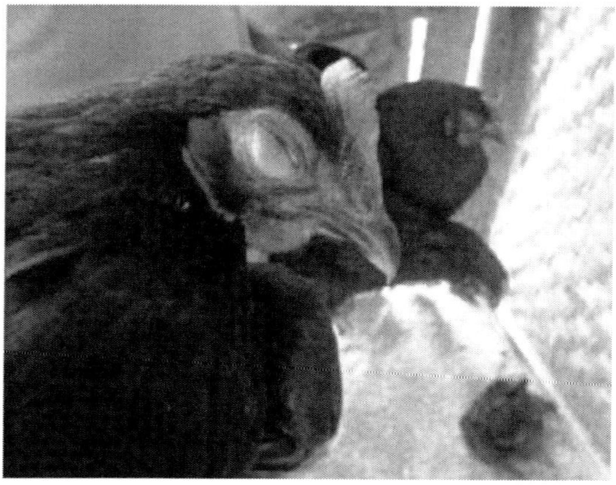

Figure 3. Typical case of swollen eyes due to NCD.

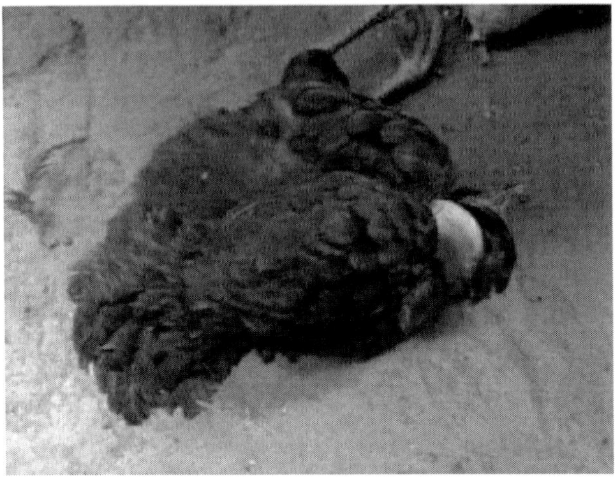

Figure 4. Typical case of torticolis in one of the affected birds with NCD.

6.4.2. Mortality

Table 8. Chicken mortalities in the treatment groups

NO	Treatment group 1 and II	Number under test per group	Mortality (%) for replicate I	Mortality (%) for replicate II
1	Infected and treated (TG3 and RG3)	18	4 (20%)	3 (20%)
2	Vaccinated with NCD and Infected NCD virus (TG5 and RG5)	18	0 (0%)	0 (0%)
3	Infected and untreated (TG2 and RG2)	18	9 (50%)	10 (60%)
4	Pretreated and infected (TG1 and RG1)	18	0 (0%)	0 (0%)
5	Uninfected and untreated (TG4 and RG4)	18	0 (0%)	0 (0%)

The infected and untreated group had up to 50% mortality in TG2 and up to 60% in RG2 while the infected and treated (TG3) group had up to 20% mortality during the observation period. There were no deaths noted among the pretreated and infected group (TG1&RG1), uninfected and untreated group (TG4&RG4) and those infected and vaccinated with NCD (TG5&RG5) Table 8.

6.4.3. Body Weights

It was observed that the body weights in the three groups i.e., infected and treated (TG3&RG3); infected and untreated (TG2&RG2) and infected and vaccinated against NCD (TG5&RG5) that had shown clinical signs decreased significantly ($p<0.05$). It was however observed that among the uninfected and untreated (TG4&RG4) and pre-treated and infected (TG1&RG1), there was insignificant weight decrease ($p>0.05$).

6.4.4. Gross Pathological Lesions

The affected chicken mostly died on day 5 post infection. The postmortem (PM) findings showed serious pathological lesions suggestive of NCD. From gross pathological examination, the carcasses showed severe conjunctivitis, facial oedema and periorbital swelling. The tracheal mucosae were severely haemorrhagic, both on upper and lower portions. Greenish intestinal content observed (Figure 6) .The proventriculi and intestinal lumen had haemorrhages (Figure 8) with button-ring like lesions in the payer's patches. The caecal tonsils were swollen (Figure 5) and the mucosae haemorrhagic. The ovaries and follicles were underdeveloped (Figure 7).

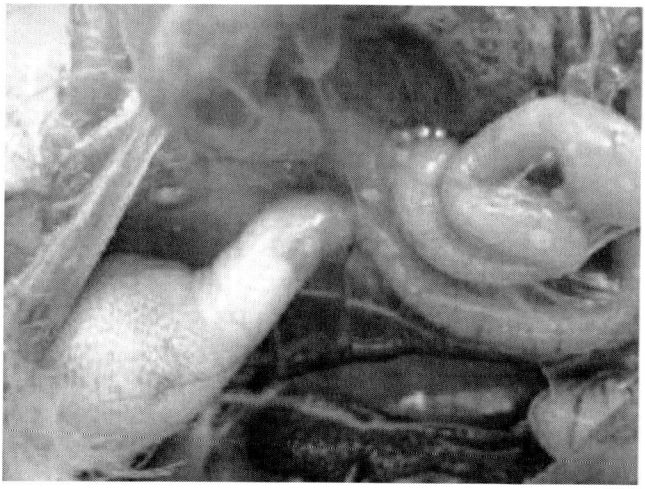

Figure 5. Swollen caecal tonsil in a case of NCD.

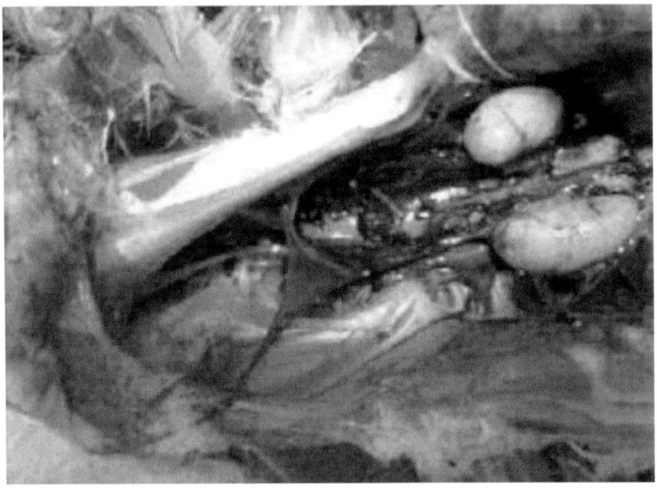

Figure 6. Greenish intestinal contents.

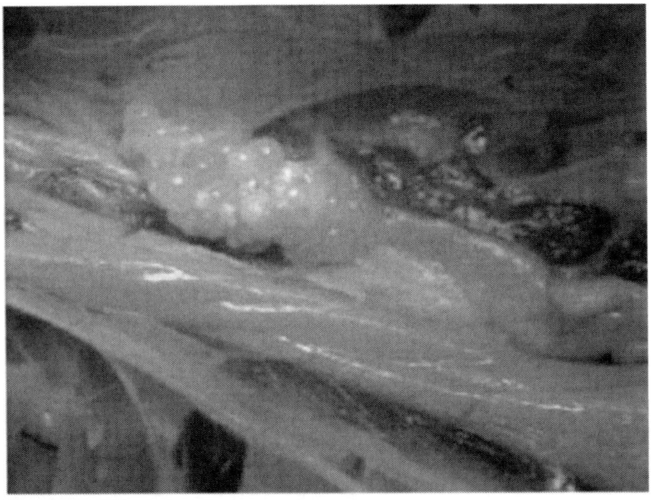

Figure 7. Under developed ovaries and follicles.

The study indicated that up to 80% of the chicken in the infected and untreated groups (TG2&RG2) had very severe lesions that varied from bird to bird in the trachea, proventriculus, intestinal lumen and ceaca. In the infected and treated groups (TG3&RG3) up to 50% of the carcasses had severe lesions. The lesions decreased in severity as the infection progressed.

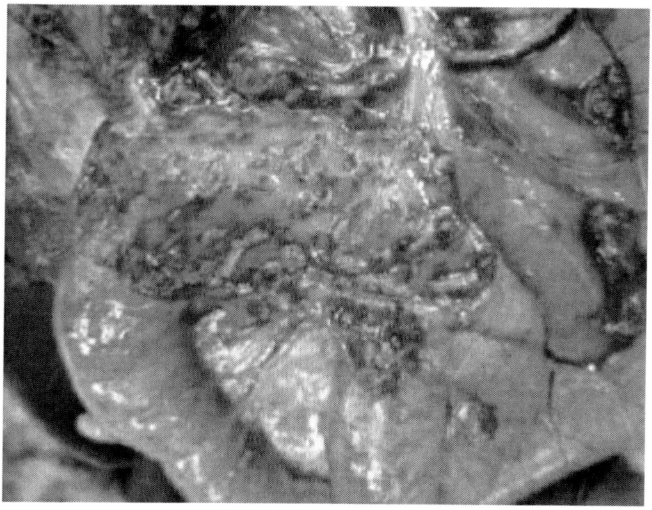

Figure 8. Severe haemorrhage in the intestinal mucosa.

6.4.5. Histopathological Lesions

There was congestion and haemorrhage in the affected heart, including massive mononuclear cell infiltration as seen in Figure 9. There were observable erosion and ulceration of the intestinal mucosa as seen in Figure 10.

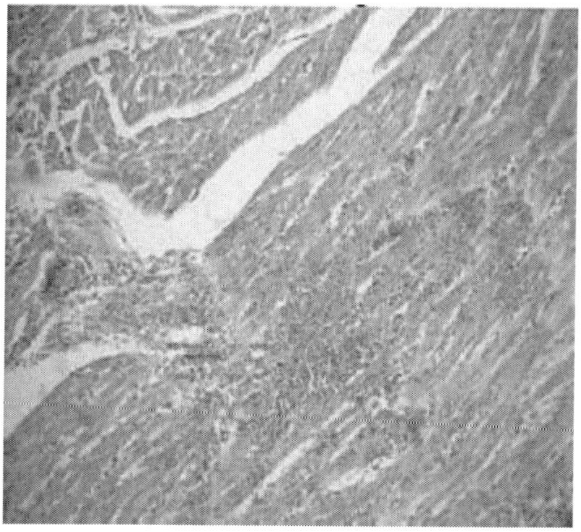

Figure 9. Masssive mononuclear cell infiltration in the heart.

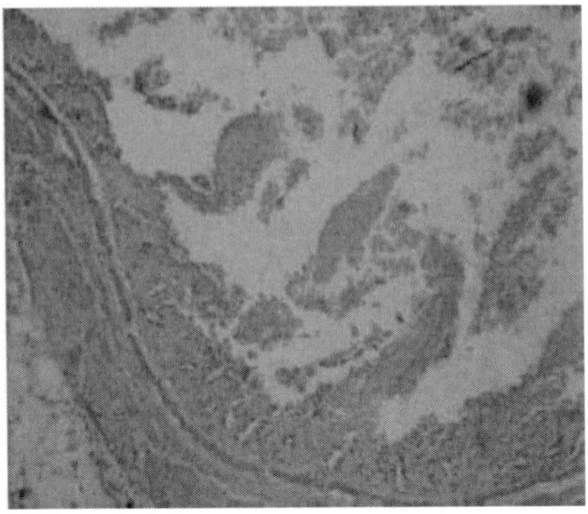

Figure 10. Intestinal ulcerative enteritis.

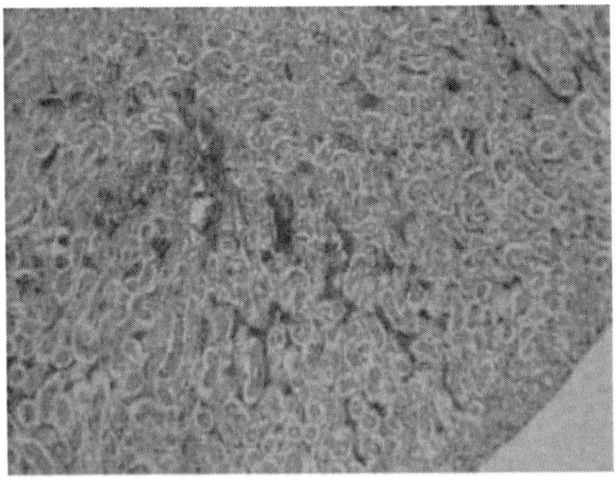

Figure 11. Fatty infiltration and haemorrhages in the kidney.

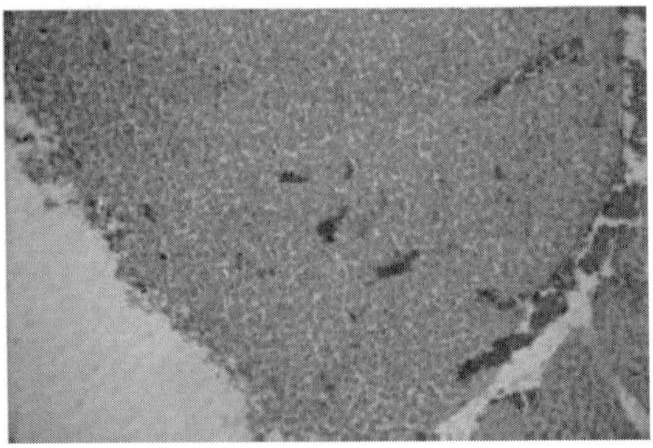

Figure 12. Liver haemorrhages.

There was haemorrhage and congestion in the kidneys; there was also perivascular necrosis and fatty infiltration of the kidney. There were observable haemorrhages in the renal cortex detailed in Figure 11. The Liver showed congestion and perivascular cuffing detailed in Figure 12.

There was severe haemorrhage, congestion and oedema in the lungs and spleen as seen in Figure 13 and 14 respectively.

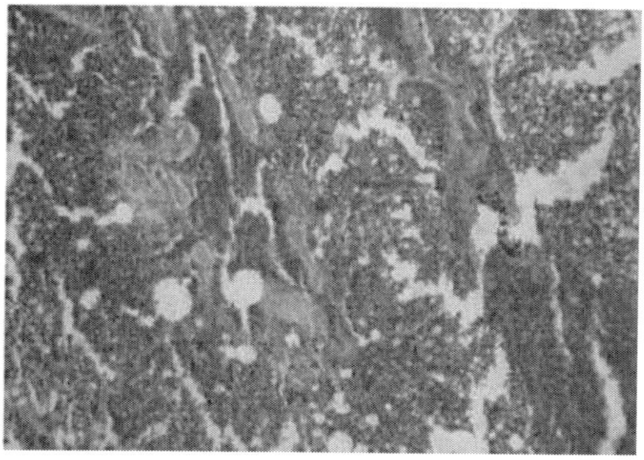

Figure 13. Lung severe haemorrhage and Oedema.

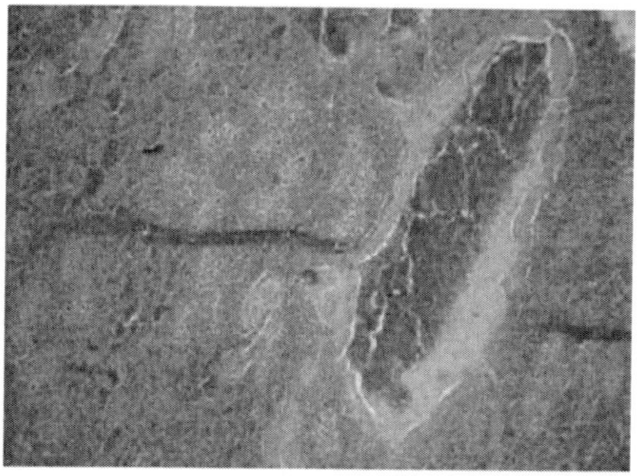

Figure 14. Spleen congestion, hemorrhage and perivascular necrosis.

6.4.6. Antibody Levels

There was generally a progressive increase in antibody titre values in all the treatment groups (Table 9). The highest being 1394.3 for infected and untreated group (TG2&RG2) followed by infected and vaccinated with NCD (TG5&RG5). Infected and treated (TG3&RG3) had up to 1066.7 titre values while pretreated and infected (TG1&RG1) attained up to 1024 titre values 22 days post infection. The lowest titre values were observed in the uninfected and untreated group (TG4&RG4) attaining 462.2 titre values.

Table 9. Tabular representation of titre values of treatment groups over one and half month period

Treatment Groups	Period of Titre Values Monitoring Over one and Half Month Period					
	Sep 21	Dec 5	Dec 9	Dec 14	Dec 27	Jan 7
Infected and treated (TG3&RG3)	12	12	616	1640	1066.7	704
Infected and vaccinated with NCD (TG5&RG5)	17	17	746.7	871.1	1208.9	657.8
Infected and untreated (TG2&RG2)	34.5	34.5	816	880	1394.3	682.5
Pre-treated and infected (TG1&RG1)	208	208	376	864	1024	1024
Uninfected and untreated (TG4&RG4)	12	12	80	208	462.2	374

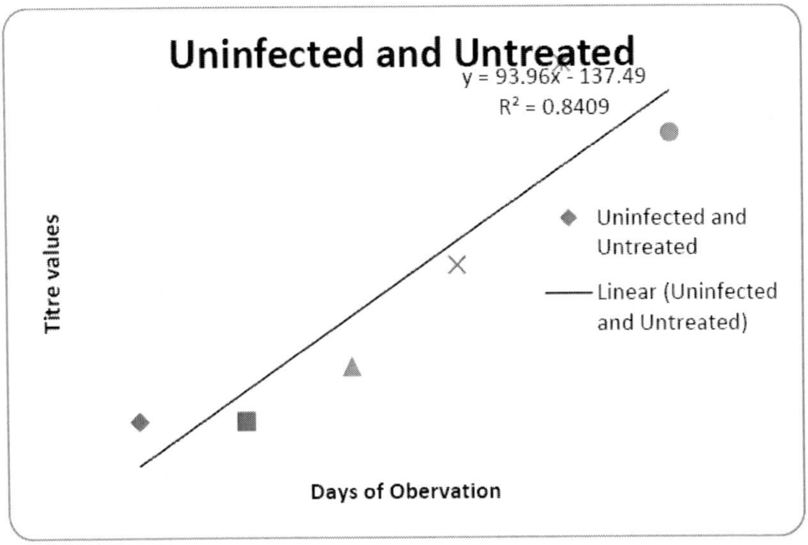

Figure 15. Titre values over a period of time among uninfected and untreated group.

The rank correlation coefficient gives a positive 84.09% relationship between the titre values and days of observation among the uninfected and untreated group (Figure 15).

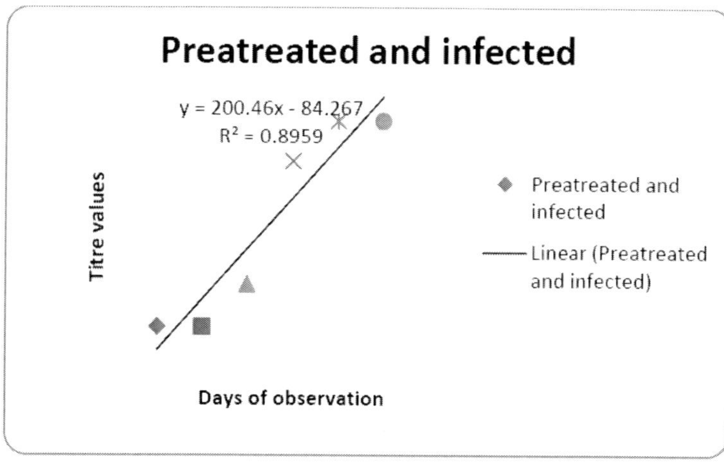

Figure 16. Antibody titre values over observation period among pre-treated, infected and treated group.

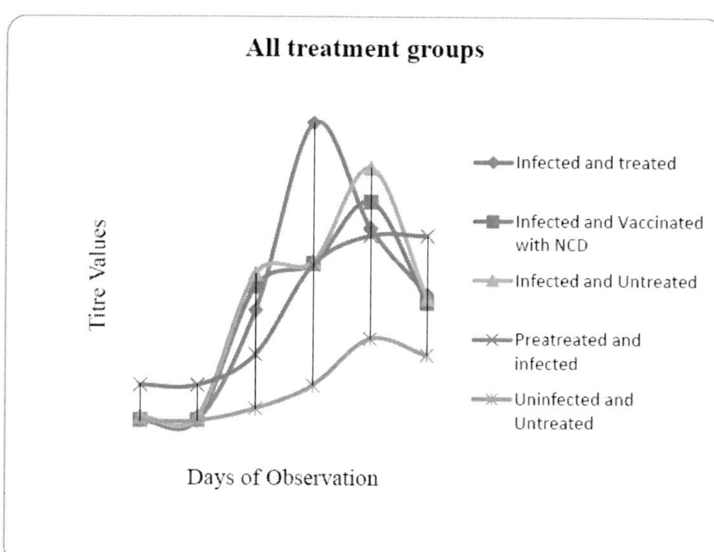

Figure 17. Titre values over observation period among pre-treated, infected and treated group.

The rank correlation coefficient gives a positive 89.59% relationship between the antibody titre values and days of observation pre-treatment, post infection and treatment among the treated group in (Figure 16).

It was observed that the uninfected and untreated group (TG4&RG4) had the lowest slope/ gradient. The highest titre attained is up to 462 titers (Figure 17). This was followed by pretreated, infected and treated (TG1&RG1) with extracts. Furthermore, the infected and vaccinated with NCD group (TG5&RG5) had a steeper slope, this was followed by infected and untreated group (TG2&RG2) and finally the infected and treated with *Capsicum annum* extracts group (TG3&RG3). The titre values decreased after 23 days (December 27th) because the body was adjusting and immune response mounted due to the antigens being contained hence the drop in tire values.

6.4.7. Haematological Results for Treatment Groups

6.4.8. Results Presentation

The haematological picture indicated that the neutrophils were within the normal range in nearly all the treatment groups with a slight increase in numbers of neutrophils among infected and treated (TG3&RG3) and pretreated and infected groups (TG1&TG2) (Table 10). Most of the lymphocytes in the treatment groups were within normal ranges except the uninfected and untreated group (TG4&RG4). Monocytes lie within the normal range. The eosinophils were higher among the uninfected and untreated (TG4&RG4) in the male birds and were also higher than normal among infected and treated (TG3&RG3) and those infected and vaccinated with NCD vaccines (TG5&RG5); pretreated and infected and treated (TG1&RG1) among females birds. The infected and untreated (TG2&RG2) and infected and treated (TG2&RG2) had normal eosinophil levels. In all the treatment groups, basophils lie within the normal ranges.

There were significant differences in haemoglobin, basophil, eosinophil levels between male and female birds ($P<0.05$). Likewise there were statistically significant differences for male and female birds ($p<0.05$) for lymphocytes, mean haemoglobin concentration (MHC), Mean Corpuscular Haemoglobin concentration (MCHC), Mean Corpuscular Volume (MCV), Monocytes, Neutrophils (NE), Platelets (PLT), Red blood cells.

Table 10. Haematological Analysis of the Treatment Groups of Indigenous Chicken

Category	Sex	NE (1.7-7.7/42-85)	LY (11-49)	MO (0-0.8/0-9)	EO(0-0.6/0-6)	BA(0-0.2/0-2)	RBC(3.8-5.30)	HGB(11-18)	HCT(36-56)	MCV (80-100)	MCH 27-32	MCHC(32-36)	RDW (10-16.5)	PLT (150-450)	MPV (5-10)
Uninfected and Untreated (TG4&RG4)	Male	28.70± 1.77	54.48± 2.23	0.146± 0.089	18.22± 0.937	0.640± 0.0809 7	3.178± 0.065	15.05± 0.255	47.15± 0.768	149± 1.04	47.48± 0.32	32.02± 0.228	10.40± 0.355	90.90± 9.487	6.780± 0.2912
	Female	27.49± 1.77	62.66± 2.23	0.458± 0.089	6.12± 0.937	1.282± 0.0809 7	2.625± 0.065	12.30± 0.255	35.26± 0.768	134.9± 1.04	44.37± 0.32	33.05± 0.228	10.56± 0.355	1.29±9 .487	8.080± 0.2912
Infected and untreated (TG2&RG2)	Male	30.20± 1.77	47.37± 2.23	1.120± 0.089	19.75± 0.937	1.450± 0.0809	2.864± 0.065	13.50± 0.255	42.98± 0.768	149.3± 1.04	47.18± 0.32	31.46± 0.228	11.33± 0.355	19.71± 9.487	9.470± 0.291
	Female	33.71± 1.77	42.41± 2.23	0.687± 0.089	16.26± 0.937	1.296± 0.0809	1.904± 0.065	10.02± 0.255	31.01± 0.768	131.7± 1.04	42.33± 0.32	32.66± 0.228	9.47± 0.355	5.23± 9.487	7.026± 0.291
Infected and treated (TG3&RG3)	Male	53.25± 1.77	32.33± 2.23	0.490± 0.089	12.29± 0.937	1.000± 0.0809	3.324± 0.065	15.74± 0.255	47.26± 0.768	142.1± 1.040± 1.04	46.42± 0.32	33.24± 0.228	10.62± 0.355	24.42± 9.487	5.740± 0.291
	Female	35.50± 1.77	46.89± 2.23	0.520± 0.089	20.47± 0.937	1.320± 0.0809	1.629± 0.065	7.68± 0.255	23.53± 0.768	134.1± 1.04	14.61± 0.32	33.30± 0.228	9.86± 0.355	6.87±9 .487	7.220± 0.291

Table 10. (Continued)

Infected and vaccinated with NCD (TG5&RG5)	Male	42.87± 1.77	41.94± 2.234	0.7740 ±0.089	9.44± 0.937	1.400± 0.0809	3.312± 0.065	16.47± 0.255	49.99± 0.768	151.2± 1.04	48.20± 0.32	33.25± 0.228	10.80± 0.355	98.20± 9.487	7.205± 0.291
	Femal	34.38± 1.77	43.89± 2.23	0.780± 0.089	17.26± 0.937	1.336± 0.0809	2.224± 0.065	10.48± 0.255	32.43± 0.768	136.3± 1.04	45.20± 0.32	33.37± 0.228	9.83± 0.355	5.42± 9.487	7.030± 0.291
Pre-treated, infected and treated (TG1& RG1)	Male	49.55± 1.77	37.91± 2.23	0.729± 0.089	6.54± 0.937	1.420± 0.0809	3.140± 0.06531	15.47± 0.255	44.42± 0.768	136.5± 1.04	45.49± 0.32	33.41± 0.228	10.00± 0.355	42.30± 9.487	5.410± 0.291
	Female	34.44± 1.77	45.81± 2.23	0.820± 0.089	18.96± 0.937	1.450± 0.0809	2.376± 0.065	10.95± 0.255	32.82± 0.768	138± 1.04	46.22± 0.32	33.36± 0.228	10.10± 0.355	4.80±9 .487	7.270± 0.291
Coefficient of variation (%)		15.11	15.50	20.92	20.39	20.33	7.77	6.31	6.28	2.34	2.21	2.19	10.92	100.29	12.93
Least significant difference (5%)		4.967	6.277	0.251	2.633	0.228	0.184	0.716	2.34	2.921	0.902	0.642	0.999	26.65	0.818

Ne=Neutrophil; Ly-Lymphocytes; Mo- Monocytes; Eo- Eosinophils; Ba- Basophils; RBC- Red Blood cells; HGB- Haemoglobin; MCV- Mean Corpuscular Volume; MCH- Mean Corpuscular haemoglobin; MCHC- Mean Corpuscular Haemoglobin concentration; PLT-Platelet.

6.4.9. Biochemical Results for Treatment Groups

The results showed that there were significant statistical differences among male and female animals ($p<0.05$) in respective to alanine phosphatase levels, creatinine levels and uric acid. There exist insignificant statistical sex difference ($P>0.05$) for aspartate levels and urea levels. It can be noted here that the alanine phosphatase and aspartate transaminase levels were higher than the normal body ranges. The alanine transaminase, creatinine, urease and uric acid were all within the normal body ranges as detailed in Table 11.

6.5. Results Discussion

The study clearly demonstrated significant clinical signs, gross lesions and histopathological signs in the infected and untreated group (TG2&RG2) and infected and treated groups (TG3&RG3), typical of signs exhibited by the viscerotropic velogenic (VV) types of Newcastle disease virus (Fi. 2-14). This is in agreement with observation by Alders and Spradbrow (2001).

Results of the post mortem examinations indicated more severe lesions among the infected and untreated groups (TG2&RG2) than pretreated and infected groups (TG1&RG1) and infected and treated groups (TG3&RG3). *Capsicum annum* exhibited antibacterial properties (Lagu and Kayanja, 2012), as well as anti-inflammatory effects. This probably exhibited prophylactic and therapeutic effects on infection by the viruses as documented by Waihenya et al. (2002). The antibodies to NCD virus in the pretreated and infected (TG1&RG1); infected and untreated (TG2&RG2) and infected and vaccinated with NCD (TG5&RG5) increased drastically over the 21 days period (Table 24). There were low titre values in the uninfected and untreated groups (TG4&RG4). Similar observations were made by (Waihenya et al., 2012). The high antibody titre values in the infected groups contribute to the recovery of some of the indigenous chicken. Cell mediated response in addition to humoral response could explain the protection in chicken that recovered from clinical cases leading to reduction in mortalities by the NCD. The antiviral effects of the extract *invivo* were probably mediated through immunomodulatory activity on macrophages leading to secretion of cytokines: Interleukines 1(IL1), interleukins 6 (IL6), Tumour necrosis factor (TNF) and interferons in agreement with the observation by Djeraba and Quere (2000). The interferon's play a protective role at the initial phases of most viral infections This would offer some protection against any viral infections a case earlier documented by Waihenya et al. (2002).

Table 11. Biochemical Analysis of the Treatment Groups

Category	Sex	ALP2L (40-129) u/l	ALTL (0-41) u/l	ASTL (0-40) u/l	CREJ2 (44-106) umol/l	UREAL (2.7-6.4) mmol/l	UA2.7-7.2 mg/dl
Infected and treated	Male	380.4±80.82	3.925±0.7126	195.8±15.88	21.65±0.9289	0.7820±0.1011	4.073±0.2246
	Female	795.9±80.82	1.829±0.7126	179.6±15.88	11.10±0.9289	0.4470±0.1011	5.290±0.2246
Infected and vaccinated with NCD	Male	599.3±80.82	2.740±0.7126	196.3±15.88	14.47±0.9289	0.6530±0.1011	4.190±0.2246
	Female	696.5±80.82	2.810±0.7126	173.2±15.88	11.70±0.9289	0.6350±0.1011	4.390±0.2246
Infected and untreated	Male	712.1±80.82	5.884±0.7126	200.0±15.88	11.20±0.9289	1.0340±0.1011	3.720±0.2246
	Female	484.8±80.82	2.950±0.7126	226.7±15.88	8.00±0.9289	0.9960±0.1011	2.430±0.2246
Pre-treated, infected and treated	Male	327.8±80.82	3.900±0.7126	199.5±15.88	22.70±0.9289	0.7940±0.1011	4.076±0.2246
	Female	759.3±80.82	3.693±0.7126	188.3±15.88	12.92±0.9289	0.8030±0.1011	3.005±0.2246
Uninfected and Untreated	Male	477.8±80.82	5.306±0.7126	159.6±15.88	9.12±0.9289	1.1250±0.1011	3.335±0.2246
	Female	851±80.82	4.486±0.7126	185.0±15.88	13.65±0.9289	0.8460±0.1011	2.530±0.2246
Coefficient of variation (%)		59.40	84.94	37.31	30.43	55.73	27.12
Least significant difference (at 5%) for predicted means		225.5	1.988	44.31	2.591	0.2821	0.6266

ALP2L- Alkaline phosphatase; ALTL- Alanine transaminase;ASTL- Aspartate transaminase; CREJ- Creatinine; UREAL- Urease; UA-Uric acid.

Hematology gives a basic knowledge on changes in blood parameters under different conditions. These conditions may be attributed to variations in life habit of the birds, nutritional status, seasonality, sex, breed, age, geographical location, climate and other important physiological factors as documented by Sharmin and Myenuddin (2004) and Albokhadaim (2012).Therefore, haematological results offer important information revealing the health status of one bird or many birds.

The Complete Blood Count (CBC) is a long-standing platform test of the clinical laboratory such WBC, RBC, Hemoglobin, Hematocrit, MCV, MCH, MCHC, Polys & Stabs, Lymphocytes, Monocytes, Basophils, Morphology, and Platelets (Smith and Hattingh, 1979).

Neutrophils were released in the circulation and blood pool as a consequence of increased activity, increased blood flow, release of epinephrine and corticosteroids, stress etc). They played important phagocytic roles and were also attracted by chemotactic stimuli and products of tissue breakdown. Increased demand for neutrophils often leads to release of immature cells into circulation (shift to the left) based upon schilling's maturation sequence.

The increase in the number of lymphocytes in this case was probably due to physiological leucocytosis and stress as suggested by Nowaczewski and Kontecka (2011).They interacted with lymphocytes (antigen processing and presentation). Monocytes were common in stress conditions, recovery stage of acute diseases, chronic suppurative diseases, diseases with considerable tissue debris and granulomatous inflammatory response Sharmin and Myenuddin (2004); Albokhadaim (2012).

Eosinophils followed the pattern of neutrophils. Act as detoxifiers, eosinophilic granules (lysosomes) contain digestive enzymes; deactivation of histamine, bradykinin, serotonin which resulted in anti-inflammatory effect also chemotactically attracted by lymphokines released by lymphocytes following antigen- antibody complexes. They contain a fibrinolytic system that assist in degradation of excessive fibrin deposits. Eosinopenia probably occured following stress and response to release of glucostereroids, stress of disease as suggested by Sharmin and Myenuddin (2004); Albokhadaim (2012).

Mean Corpuscular Volume (MCV) is an indication of the size of the red cells. In this study, overall the MCV values were higher than the normal ranges of 80 fl- 100 fl, a situation described as macrocytic cells. Mean Corpuscular Hemoglobin (MCH) is a measure of the amount of hemoglobin per red blood cell; in this study most of the hemoglobin per red blood cells was higher than the range of 27 pg-32 pg except in the female chicken, infected and treated group where the MCH was 14.61 pg. It should be noted here that true hyperchromic cells do not exist. However, cells larger than normal may contain quantitatively larger amounts of hemoglobin than are found in normal cells. The larger cells in these groups may be due to physiological stress since they are housed in the experimental units under non free range movements.

The biochemical analysis of the liver function enzymes and kidney function tests (Table 26) showed that the alkaline phosphatase levels were much higher than the normal range of (40-129) u/l; alanine transaminase levels were generally within the normal range of (0-41) u/l; aspartate transaminase were higher than the normal ranges of (0-40) u/l in all the treatment groups; creatinine in all the treatment groups were lower than the normal range of (44-106) umol/l; Urease levels in all the treatment groups were below the expected normal values of (2.7-6.4) mmol/ as was also noted by Abdi-Hachesco, Talebi and Asri-Rezaei (2011), Simaraks et al. (2004), Chinrasri and Aengwanich (2007). While, uric acid levels in all the treatment groups were within the normal range of (2.7-7.2) mg/dl indicating minimal disturbances with the kidney functions in agreement with the findings by Chandra et al. (2010).

Alkaline phosphatase (ALP) catalyzes the hydrolysis of phosphate esters in alkaline buffer and produces an organic radical and inorganic phosphate. Changes in alkaline phosphatase level and activity are associated with various disease states in the liver and bone (Abdi-Hachesco et al., 2011).

Alanine transaminase (ALAT) is also called serum glutamic pyruvic transaminase (SGPT) or alanine aminotransferase (ALT). ALT is found in serum and in various bodily tissues, but is usually associated with the liver. It catalyzes the reaction: α-ketoglutarate + alanine ⇋ glutamate + pyruvate. It is commonly measured clinically as a part of a diagnostic liver function test to determine liver health. Diagnostically, it is almost always measured in units/liter (U/L).

Aspartate transaminase (AST), also called aspartate aminotransferase (AspAT/ASAT/AAT) or serum glutamic oxaloacetic transaminase (SGOT) is a pyridoxal phosphate (PLP)-dependent transaminase enzyme. AST catalyzes the reversible transfer of an α-amino group between aspartate and glutamate and, as such, is an important enzyme in amino acid metabolism. AST is found in the liver, heart, skeletal muscle, kidneys, brain, and red blood cells, and is commonly measured clinically as a marker for liver health. Aspartate transaminase catalyzes the interconversion of aspartate and α-ketoglutarate to oxaloacetate and glutamate.

AST is similar to alanine transaminase (ALT) in that both enzymes are associated with liver parenchymal cells. The difference is that ALT is found predominantly in the liver, with clinically negligible quantities found in the kidneys, heart, and skeletal muscle, while AST is found in the liver, heart (cardiac muscle), skeletal muscle, kidneys, brain, and red blood cells. As a result, ALT is a more specific indicator of liver inflammation than AST, as AST may be elevated also in diseases affecting other organs, such as myocardial infarction, acute pancreatitis, acute hemolytic anemia, severe burns, acute renal disease, musculoskeletal diseases, and trauma.

AST was defined as a biochemical marker for the diagnosis of acute myocardial infarction. However, the use of AST for such a diagnosis is now redundant and has been superseded by the cardiac troponins. AST (SGOT) is commonly measured clinically as a part of diagnostic liver function tests, to determine liver health.

Major routes of creatinine (Cr) metabolism in the mammalian body. The most part (up to 94%) of Cr is found in muscular tissues. Because muscle has virtually no Cr-synthesizing capacity, Cr has to be taken up from the blood against a large concentration gradient by a saturable, Na^+- and Cl^--dependent Cr transporter that spans the plasma membrane (Li et al., 2010). The daily demand for Cr is met either by intestinal absorption of dietary Cr or by de novo Cr biosynthesis. The first step of Cr biosynthesis probably occurs mainly in the kidney, whereas the liver is likely to be the principal organ accomplishing the subsequent methylation of guanidinoacetic acid (GAA) to Cr. It must be stressed that the detailed contribution of different bodily tissues (pancreas, kidney, liver, testis) to total Cr synthesis is still rather unclear and may vary between species (Li et al., 2010). The muscular Cr and PCr are nonenzymatically converted at an almost steady rate (~2% of total Cr per day) to creatinine (Crn), which diffuses out of the cells and is excreted by the kidneys into the urine.

Creatinine is commonly measured in urine and is a key benchmark for the normalization of a variety of urinary biomarkers. Serum creatinine levels, however, are a useful indicator of renal function. In addition, abnormal creatinine levels have been implicated in diabetes, cardiovascular, and circulatory diseases. Cayman's Creatinine (serum) Assay is designed to measure creatinine levels in plasma and serum. The assay relies on the Jaffe' reaction, where in a yellow/orange color forms when the metabolite is treated with alkaline picrate. The rate of color development is directly proportional to the concentration of creatinine in the sample and is measured at an absorbance between 490-500 nm. The kinetic nature of the assay eliminates interference from extraneous serum contaminants, such as lipids and bilirubin.

The enzyme urease enhances the rate of urea hydrolysis at pH 8.0 and 20 ^{0}C by a factor of 10. If a given quantity of urease can completely hydrolyze a given quantity of urea in 5.0 min at 20 ^{0}C and pH 8.0, how long would it take for this amount of urea to be hydrolyzed under the same conditions in the absence of urease.

Uric acid is a heterocyclic compound of carbon, nitrogen, oxygen, and hydrogen with the formula $C_5H_4N_4O_3$. It forms ions and salts known as urates and acid urates such as ammonium acid urate. Uric acid is a product of the metabolic breakdown of purine nucleotides. In birds uric acid also is the end product of purine metabolism, but it is excreted in feces as a dry mass. This involves a complex metabolic pathway that is energetically costly in comparison to processing of other nitrogenous wastes such as urea (from urea cycle) or ammonia, but has the advantage of reducing water loss. It should be observed that the catabolism of nitrogen gives uric acid. The nutritional status, sex and age may influence the levels of blood uric in birds an issue agreed by Albokhadaim (2012).

CONCLUSION AND RECOMMENDATIONS

Capsicum annum is a very useful herbal medicine that can be used to control the outbreak of Newcastle disease. The use of *C. annum* must follow right concentration, dose and standards in mixing the extracts. The extracts should be pre administered (prophylactic treatment) before the outbreak of the NCD. Alcohol extracts performed better than aqueous extracts. In groups especially the infected and untreated (TG2&RG2), there was up to 60% mortality in the affected groups. For the infected groups, it was clear that NCD was a big problem to the farmers. Prophylactic treatment with *C. annum* (TG1&RG1) by at least one week before infection reduces mortality by over 90%.

The conventional approaches to vaccinate the birds using thermo-labile and thermo-stable vaccines still works except its access and use among peasant farmers is still problematic and limited because of the small sizes of chicken per households. The clinical signs, gross lesions, histopathology, serology all indicated presence of NCD in the infected and treated group (TG3&RG3). It was clear that *C. annum* extracts were not very dangerous to the liver and kidneys as per the liver and kidney function tests done. The study revealed that with increasing time post viral inoculation in the test birds, the antibody titres correspondingly increased drastically hence offering solid immunity. The study recommends farmer friendly packages developed to guide farmers in the administration of the herbal *C. annum* concoctions and their popularization.

Chapter 7

IN VIVO EFFICACY OF *ERYTHRINA ABYSSINICA* ON *ASCARIDIA GALLI* AND COMMON INTERNAL PARASITES IN INDIGENOUS CHICKEN

ABSTRACT

Erythrina abyssinica was efficacious in the control of *Ascaridia galli*. It was also effective in the control of *Trychostrongylus tenuis* and coccidian parasites to a certain degree. Generally, haematological and biochemical tests revealed very minimum disturbances in the liver and kidney functions. It can therefore be concluded that, it is safe to use *E. abyssinica* leaf extracts in the control of *Ascaridia galli* infections, *Trychostrongylus tenuis* and coccidian parasites. Cases of reinfection for the case of coccidian species are very common phenomena.

The efficacy of *E. abyssinica* is comparable to the conventional drug Piperazine citrate. Piperazine citrate is ineffective in the control of coccidia infections. The relationship between the treatment groups and egg per gram reduction was expressed in correlation rank coefficient (r^2) ranged from *E. abyssinica* leaves extracts (95.09%), Piperazine citrate (92.56%) and negative control (95.43%).

Further understanding of the bioactive compounds responsible for activity against the parasites was vital. It is also important to undertake sub acute and chronic toxicity studies. Thc study further recommended appropriate simple, user friendly standardization of the E. abyssinica leaf extracts for farmers to use.

7.1. Introduction

Indigenous chicken are sold to meet household needs like school fees, medical expenses, clothings etc. Indigenous chicken are active in pest control (Alders and Pym, 2009). They are required for social functions and their faecal droppings are sources of manure for improving yields for crops.

Most indigenous chicken are kept in free range hence are faced with numerous worm and internal parasite infestations. The indigenous chickens receive minimal drug application to control the various infestations and hence they are burdened by the internal parasites (Tolossa et al., 2009). A big number of the rural folk use herbal concoctions to control *Ascaridia galli* infections and other internal parasites. One of these herbal concoctions is from *E. abyssinica* leaf and root bark extracts.

The role of *Erythrina abyssinica* in the management of *Ascaridia galli* and common internal parasites is well documented (ITDG and IIRR 1996; Lagu and Kayanja, 2010 and Lagu and Kayanja, 2013).

It is not clear how effective the *Erythrina abyssinica* extracts are against *Ascaridia galli* and the common internal parasites affecting the free range indigenous chicken. The herbal formulations are not standardized and are used in various dosages (Street et al., 2008). This study hypothesized that *Erythrina abyssinica* leaf extracts is effective in the control of helminths among the indigenous chicken.

The study aim was to determine the effectiveness of *Erythrina abyssinca* leaves extracts in the control of *Ascaridia galli* and internal parasites in indigenous chicken.

7.2. Materials and Methods

7.2.1. Study Design

The leaves extracts of *Erythrina abyssinica* were collected from Mbarara district. A randomized controlled trial was used in the study. The trial had E. abyssinica leaves extracts as test sample, Piperazine citrate as positive control and distilled water as negative control. The selected birds were randomly allocated to the different treatment groups.

7.2.2. Selection Criteria

The study plant was selected basing on the fact that, *invitro* studies were conducted on efficacy of plant parts and the leaves were found to exhibit activity on the *Ascaridia galli* (Lagu and Kayanja, 2013).

7.2.3. Plant Collection and Identification

The leaves of *E. abyssinica* were harvested and the collected specimens were identified at the Department of Biology, Mbarara University of Science and Technology Voucher specimen (Ea 001Lag) was prepared and kept at the Mbarara University of Science and Technology Herbarium.

7.2.4. Drying and Pulverization

The plant leaves were dried under shade at MbaZARDI, to avoid direct sunshine that could degrade some of the compounds in the plants (Bunalema et al., 2011). They were also turned over regularly, to avoid fermenting and rotting. The drying process took at least 14 days. The dried parts were then pulverized using a motor and pestle, the powder weighed using an analytical scale, and stored at room temperature.

7.2.5. Extract Preparation

250 g of freshly dried powdered leaves were macerated in 2000 ml of 70% ethanol for 72 hours with intermittent shaking. Filtration through cotton wool was done to remove coarse particles (residues) followed by filter paper 12.5 mm (Whitman®, No.1).

The filtrate was concentrated on rota-vapour under reduced pressure at 40^0C. The concentrated extracts were later dried on weighed kidney dishes to a constant weight at 50^0C. The dried extracts were packed into universal bottles and kept at 4^0C until needed for bioassays.

7.2.6. Chicken Rearing and Identification

The experimental chicken were bought at one day old and reared till the age of 4 months at Ruharo ward, Mbarara Municipality. The birds were housed and routinely released to scavenge outside the housing unit similar to the indigenous chickens kept on free range. The birds mixed freely with other chickens in the neighbourhood. No deworming was undertaken during the rearing period. The birds naturally acquired infection during the normal routine scavenging. All the birds under study were all wing tagged using modified plastic tags locally made by the researcher. The identification numbers were recorded in a counter book and chicken age, weight, sex noted and color described.

7.2.7. Experimental Design

A total of thirty five birds per treatment group in two replicates were allocated to three treatment groups namely *Erythrina abyssinica* extract group (T1&R1), *Piperazine citrate* group (positive control) (T2&R2)) and negative control group (T3&R3). The birds were kept in different compartments for the two replicates. The compartments were purposely designed for the study experiment and clearly labelled as per trial groups. The birds during the experimental trials were fed using formulated feeds and given clean water *adlibitum* and were kept inside the compartments within the poultry house. The formulated feeds lack dewormers. This was to ensure that the birds did not get access to extraneous materials in the environment which would affect the outcomes of the study. The trial was run for a period of one month from 11th November 2012 to 13th December 2012.

7.2.8. Faecal and Blood Sampling and Storage

All the faecal samples were collected by placing the birds humanely for at least 4 hours in a highly ventilated comfortable gunny bag till they defecated. The fresh faecal droppings were picked every morning and placed in a labelled and identified specimen bottles and kept in a cool box. At Mbarara specialist's diagnostic laboratory the faecal material was examined using the McMaster technique for egg per gram (epg) determination.

The wing vein sites were disinfected with iodine solution to prevent contamination and infection. The blood samples were collected from wing veins of the experiemental chicken using a sterile needle both in specimen tubes without anticoagulant and those with coagulant (EDTA). The collected blood samples were kept in a cool box and taken to central laboratory of college of Veterinary Medicine Animal Resources and Biosecurity (COVAB), Makerere University for analysis. For haematological tests using White blood cell counter machine (automatic counter Sysmex, K21. Tokyo, Japan) whole blood in vacutainers with EDTA was used. For biochemical analysis, serum was used to undertake liver and kidney function tests using an automated analytical machine and Liver function test machine (COBAS INTEGRA 400, Germany).

7.2.9. Preparation of Piperazine Citrate Stock Solution

A 100% *Piperazine citrate* powder was bought from a known Veterinary pharmacy in Kampala. Of this 30 gm were weighed and dissolved in 600 mls of Goodwin's solution to make a stock solution of 50 mg/ml of the drug as the highest concentrated dose level. The stock concentration was then serially diluted to make final concentrations as per the weight of the birds for the experiment.

7.2.10. Preparation of *Erythrina Abyssinica* Leaf Extracts for Administration

The method for *Erythrina abyssinica* leaves extraction and standardization has been described in Chapter 7 subsection 7.2.3 to 7.2.5 of this book.. The formular for calculating doses was according to body weight of the bird, within the body weights of 1.9- 4 kg.

For a stock solution of 100 mg/ml, a quarter (1/4) of the lethal dose (LD50) was obtained as the highest dose, then the dosage volume as per bird was calculated as follows, taking into account a bird of 1.9 kg;

Vol (ml)= bodyweight(kg) x dose rate(mg/kg)/stock concentration(mg/ml) equation vi;

Vol (mls) = 1.9 kg*759.81/100=14.43 ml, therefore this bird of the weight 1.9 kg is supposed to take a volume of 14.43mls of the prepared crude *Erythrina abyssinica* extracts.

This formula was reciprocated to calculate the dose to be administered to the rest of the birds in the experimental group.

7.2.11. McMaster Egg Counting Technique

This is another method of determining the number of nematode eggs per gram of faeces in order to estimate the worm burden in an animal. The advantage of this method is that, it is quick as the eggs are floated free of debris before counting.

About 4 grams of fresh faecal sample was weighed and placed into a container and 56 ml of saturated sodium chloride (NaCl) was added as flotation fluid. The contents of the beaker where stirred thoroughly with a fork, tongue depressor or spatula. The faecal suspension was filtered through a tea strainer or double layer of cheesecloth or dental napkin into the second container.

The filtrate was stirred and during this action a sub-sample was withdrawn with a pasteur pipette as the filtrate was being stirred. Faeces may contain hazardous pathogens (bacteria, viruses etc) therefore appropriate hygiene and safety procedures were employed. Local health and safety regulations were observed. The fluid was stirred and the first compartment of the McMaster counting chamber was filled with the sub sample. The fluid was stirred again and the second chamber was filled with another sub sample. The counting chamber was allowed to stand for 5 minutes. It was important to leave the chamber to stand to allow the eggs to float to the surface and the debris to go to the bottom of the chamber. The subsample of the filtrate was examined under the compound microscope at 10 x 10 magnifications. It was not necessary to use higher magnification.

All the eggs were identified and eggs within the engraved area of both chambers counted.

The numbers of eggs per gram were calculated as follows:

- Counted all the number of eggs within the grid of each chamber, ignoring those outside the squares
- Multiplied all the total by 50 – this gave the eggs per gram of faeces (e.p.g.)

For example:

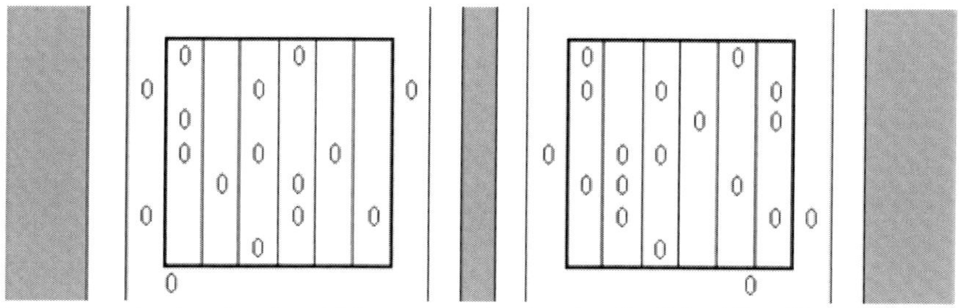

12 eggs seen in chamber 1 and 15 eggs seen in chamber 2= (12 +15) x 50 = 1350 e.p.g.

It was important to ensure that there was no delay in reading the count beyond the recommended time, as the flotation fluid could have distorted or destroyed delicate eggs. Therefore, only a few samples were processed at a time. The detailed life cycle of *Ascaridia galli*, *Trichostrongylus tenuis*and Coccidia species are well described by Georgi (1980) and Urquhart et al. (1996).

Haematological and Biochemical Analysis of Blood Samples

The haematological and biochemical analysis of blood samples were done using the automatic recording machines i.e., white blood cell counter machine (automatic counter Sysmex, K21, Tokyo, Japan) and Liver function test machine (COBAS INTEGRA 400, Germany).

7.3. DATA ANALYSIS

Data was entered in Microsoft Excel windows 2007. It was exported to Genstat Discovery Edition version 14.1 (Gentat, 2011) where Analysis of Variance was conducted with unbalanced designs. The Cofficient of variation, means, least significance difference at 5% level was analyzed. The summary data of the results were then tabulated. Paired t-test was conducted for comparison of two equal sized sets of data.

Graphical analysis and representation of data was done using Micro-soft EXCEL program. The results of clinical signs and mortality rates, body weights, pathological lesions, antibody levels was summarized and discussed holistically to represent the efficacy of *Erythrina abyssinica* among local chicken.

Table 12. Egg per Gram in the Treatment Groups

				Ascaridia galli					*Trichostronglus species*					Coccidia				
Sex	EA EXTRACT	Dose (mg/kg body wt)	Av. Weight (kg)	11-Nov	22-Nov	29-Nov	6-Dec	13-Dec	11-Nov	22-Nov	29-Nov	6-Dec	13-Dec	11-Nov	22-Nov	29-Nov	6-Dec	13-Dec
Male	NEGATIVE CONTROL (T3&R3)	0	2.1	135	150	220	256	295	110	265	320	400	485	300	500	650	790	880
Female	NEGATIVE CONTROL (T3&R3)	0	1.91	150	175	225	275	340	200	315	390	415	510	175	325	390	470	580
Male	Erythrina EXTRACT (T1&R1)	1470	2.1	450	200	100	50	50	365	350	215	190	170	1170	385	200	780	500
Female	Erythrina EXTRACT (T1&R1)	1470	1.91	300	250	150	100	50	425	225	115	90	275	450	100	175	250	150
Male	PIPERAZINE (T2&T2)	1000	2.1	200	100	70	50	50	305	300	235	200	250	165	255	300	310	315
Female	PIPERAZINE (T2&R2)	1000	1.91	180	130	80	40	40	285	385	315	175	450	725	885	975	1125	1140

This Table shows the egg per gram for treatment groups viz; negative control (T3&R3), *Erythrina abyssinica* (T1&R1) administered 1470 mg/kg body weight per bird and *Piperazine citrate* (T2&R2) given 1000 mg/kg body weight per bird. Males and female birds have weight differences by 100 grams. Generally the egg per gram for negative control increased steadily while for the extracts and piperazine reduced drastically.

7.4. Results

7.4.1. Effects of the various extracts on *Ascaridia galli* and other internal parasites

Generally, *Piperazine citrate* (T2&R2) and *Erythrina abyssinica* (T1&R1) leaf extract caused a systematic reduction in parasite egg per gram post administration of the drug and herbal concoctions till day 28 of the observation period (Figure 18) whereas negative control (T3&R3) had no effect on egg per gram reduction. The correlation rank coefficient (r^2) for the negative control (T3&R3) is (95.43%); *Piperazine citrate* (T2&R2) (92.56%) and *Erythrina abyssinica* (T1&R1) is 95.09%.

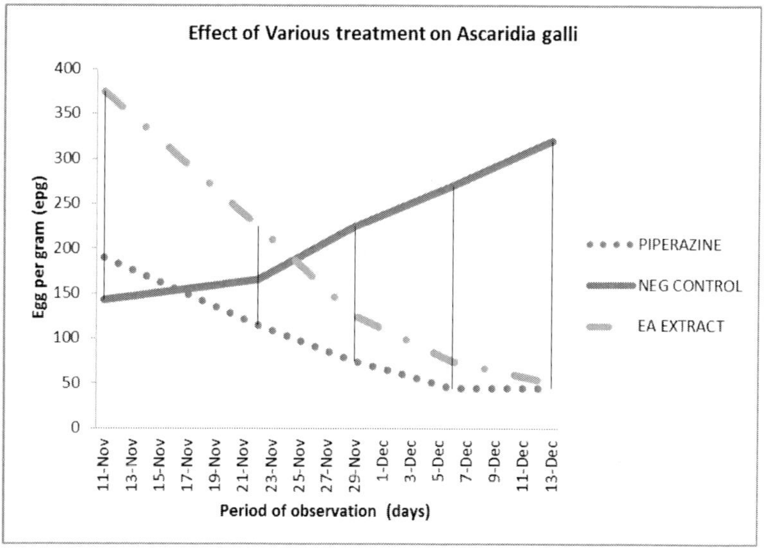

Figure 18. Shows the efficacy of different treatments on *Ascaridia galli*.

7.4.2. Efficacy of Various Treatments on *Trichostrongylus*

Figure 19 illustrates the various effects of *Erythrina abyssinica* leaves extracts (T1&R1), *Piperazine citrate* (T2&R2) and negative control (T3&R3) on *Trichostrogylus tenuis*. Generally there was reduction in egg per gram due to the effects of *Erythrina abyssinica* leaves extracts (T1&R1), *Piperazine citrate* (T2&R2) till 26 days post treatment when the eggs per gram begun to rise again. The correlation rank coefficient (r^2) for the negative control (T3&R3) was (95.43%); *Piperazine citrate* (T2&R2*)* (92.56%) and *Erythrina abyssinica* (T1&R1), 95.09%.

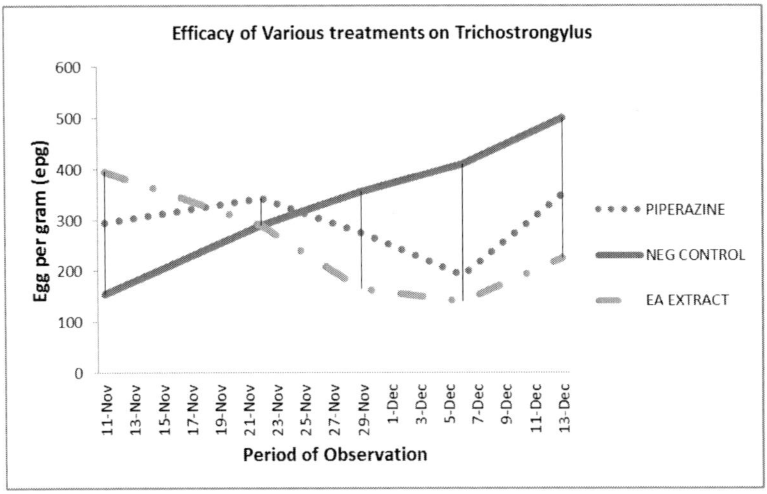

Figure 19. Efficacy of various treatments on *Trichostrongylus.*

7.4.3. Efficacy of Various Treatments on Coccidia

The efficacy of *Piperazine citrate* (T2&R2), *Erythrina abyssinica* (T1&R1) and negative control (T3&R3) is as illustrated in Figure 20. Generally, *Piperazine citrate* (T2&R2) and negative control (T3&R3) had no effect on parasite egg per gram load as seen by the steady rise in egg numbers. There was significant parasite egg per gram reduction for 19 days post treatment. Then the egg per gram begun to rise again for another 7 days then fell down again. The correlation rank coefficient (r^2) for the negative control (T3&R3) is (95.43%); *Piperazine citrate* (T2&R2 (92.56%) and *Erythrina abyssinica* (T1&R1) is 95.09%.

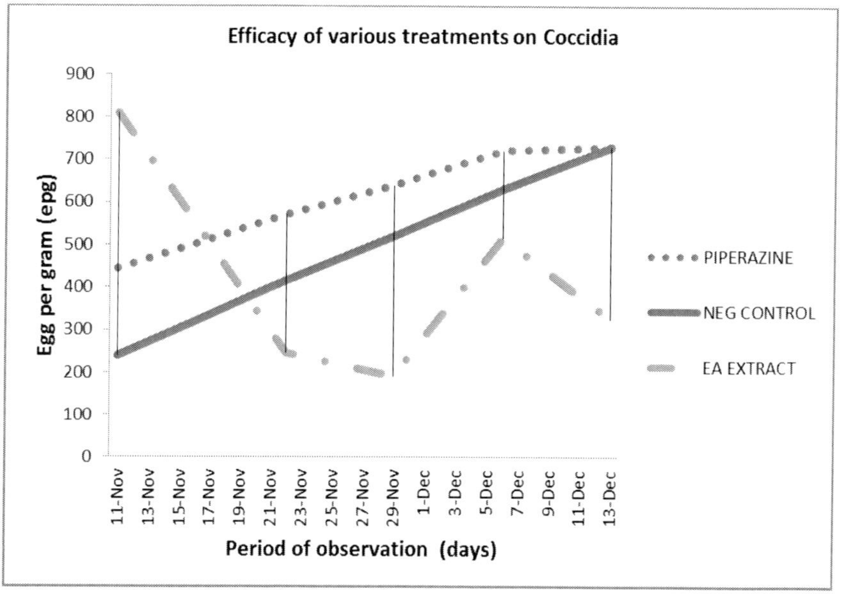

Figure 20. Efficacy of various treatments on Coccidia.

7.4.4. Haematological results for Treatment groups

Results

There were statistically significant differences between male and female birds ($p<0.05$) for blood parameters Eosinophils, haemoglobin, lymphocytes. Additionally, there were significant sex differences ($P<0.05$) for Mean corpuscular volume (MCV), monocytes, neutrophils, Red blood cells and white blood cells.

It was however, noted that there were insignificant sex differences ($P>0.05$) for parameters Mean Corpuscular Haemoglobin Concentration (MCHC) and Mean Concentration Volume (MCV).

Generally, it is observed in Table 13 that neutrophils fall within the normal range. Lymphocytes were slightly above the normal values except in the treatment group for *Erythrina abyssinica (T1&R1)* male; negative control (T3&R3) female chicken and *Piperazine citrate* (T2&R2) female. Monocytes, basophils, Red blood cells and haemoglobin had normal ranges. MCV lied above the normal range of (80-100) and MCHC (32-26) Table 13.

Table 13. Haematological analysis of the treatment groups

Category	Sex	NE(1.7-7.7/42-85)	LY(0.4-4.4/11-49)	MO (0-0.8/0-9)	EO(0-0.6/0-6)	BA(0-0.2/0-2)	RBC(3.8-5.30)	HGB(11-18)	HCT(36-56)	MCV(80-100)	MCH 27-32	MCHC(32-36)	RDW(10-16.5)	PLT(150-450)	MPV(5-10)
Erythrina abyssinica (T1&R1)	Male	10.83± 1.154	70.25± 3.903	0.2730± 0.02641	8.38± 1.226	1.6100± 0.1005	3.013± 0.1447	16.96± 0.8499	43.93± 2.327	137.9± 2.681	66.93± 4.044	42.68± 3.275	25.63± 2.562	16± 14.58	7.900± 0.2103
	Female	14.01± 1.154	44.77± 3.903	0.3020± 0.02641	23.06± 1.226	0.1650± 0.1005	2.677± 0.1447	15.96± 0.8499	37.04± 2.327	138.4± 2.681	66.82± 4.044	47.06± 3.275	20.52± 2.431	87± 14.58	6.850± 0.2103
Negative Control (T3&R3)	Male	16.45± 1.154	39.58± 3.903	0.3600± 0.02641	62.41± 1.226	0.0600± 0.1005	1.808± 0.1447	11.72± 0.8499	25.10± 2.327	144± 2.681	60.36± 4.044	43.26± 3.275	11.78± 2.431	17.80± 14.58	8.600± 0.2103
	Female	10.19± 1.154	68.04± 3.903	0.1950± 0.02641	10.46± 1.226	0.5000± 0.1005	3.165± 0.1447	19.29± 0.8499	43.46± 2.327	136.2± 2.681	59.15± 4.044	47.04± 3.275	17.27± 2.431	102± 14.58	7.620± 0.2103
Piperazine citrate (T2&R2)	Male	1.49± 1.154	44.97± 3.903	0.0470± 0.02641	28.42± 1.226	0.0700± 0.1005	1.580± 0.1447	9.96± 0.8499	22.27± 2.327	132± 2.681	75.06± 4.044	55.68± 3.275	16.02± 2.431	47.60± 14.58	12.020 ± 0.2103

Category	Sex	NE(1.7-7.7/42-85)	LY(0.4-4.4/11-49)	MO (0-0.8/0-9)	EO(0-0.6/0-6)	BA(0-0.2/0-2)	RBC(3.8-5.30)	HGB(11-18)	HCT(36-56)	MCV(80-100)	MCH 27-32	MCHC(32-36)	RDW(10-16.5)	PLT(150-450)	MPV(5-10)
	Female	15.78± 1.154	57.77± 3.903	0.2850± 0.02641	22.61± 1.226	0.6900± 0.1005	3.085± 0.1447	16.57± 0.8499	41.32± 2.327	133± 2.681	55.02± 4.044	44.92± 3.275	12.56± 2.431	128.10 ± 14.58	7.440± 0.2103
Least Significant Difference		3.233	10.93	0.0074	3.44	0.28	0.41	2.38	6.52	7.51	11.33	9.17	6.81	40.86	0.59
Coefficient of variation (%)		45.05	32.18	48.46	21.19	87.11	25.32	25.21	29.30	8.76	28.30	31.31	63.37	98.12	11.19

Ne=Neutrophil; Ly-Lymphocytes; Mo- Monocytes; Eo- Eosinophils; Ba- Basophils; RBC- Red Blood cells; HGB- Haemoglobin; MCV- Mean Corpuscular Volume; MCH- Mean Corpuscular haemoglobin; MCHC- Mean Corpuscular Haemoglobin concentration; PLT-Platelets.

Table 14. Biochemical analysis of the treatment groups

Category	Sex	ALP2L (40-129)u/l	ALTL (0-41) u/l	ASTL (0-40) u/l	CREJ2 (44-106) umol/l	UREAL (2.7-6.4) mmol/l	UA 2.7-7.2mg/dl
Erythrina abyssinica (T1&R1)	Male	609.3±38.74	2.750±0.1820	206.3±9.309	11.500±0.5594	0.4800±0.02215	1.230±0.04351
	Female	619.9±38.74	1.860±0.1820	152.7±9.309	8.200±0.5594	0.4300±0.02215	1.420±0.04351
Negative Control (T3&R3)	Male	652.7±38.74	2.420±0.1820	216.1±9.309	7.750±0.5594	0.4600±0.02215	1.200±0.04351
	Female	619.9±38.74	1.790±0.1820	154.1±9.309	8.160±0.5594	0.5200±0.02215	1.680±0.04351
Piperazine citrate (T2&R2)	Male	540.2±38.74	1.860±0.1820	193.5±9.309	8.240±0.5594	0.5000±0.02215	0.800±0.04351
	Female	594.9±38.74	2.210±0.1820	154.2±9.309	11.400±0.5594	0.4430±0.02215	1.450±0.04351
Least Significant difference		108.5	0.5099	26.08	1.567	0.06205	0.1219
Coefficient of variation (%cv)		28.58	37.89	23.20	27.17	20.98	15.01

ALP2L- Alkaline phosphatase; ALTL- Alanine transaminase; ASTL- Aspartate transaminase; CREJ- Creatinine; UREAL- Urease; UA-Uric acid.

7.4.5. Biochemical Results for Treatment Groups of Indigenous Chicken

Table 14 illustrates the Biochemical analysis of the treatment groups viz; *Erythrina abyssinica (T1&R1)*, *Piperazine citrate (T2&R2)* and Negative Control (T3&R3). The following parameters were analysed *Alkaline phosphatase* (ALP2L); *Alanine transaminase* (ALTL); *Aspartate transaminase* (ASTL); Creatinine (CREJ); Urease (UREAL); Uric acid (UA). The results showed that *Alkaline phosphatase* (ALP2L) had higher figures than normal values of (40-129) u/l. *Alanine transaminase* (ALTL) lies within the normal values. *Aspartate transaminase* (ASTL) lies above the normal values of (0-40)u/l; Creatinine (CREJ), Urease (UREAL) and Uric acid (UA) all have slightly below the expected normal values.

7.5. Discussions of Results

Overall, there were drastic and steady decline in egg per gram due to effects of *Erythrina abyssinica* and *Piperazine citrate* on *Ascaridia galli, Trichostronglus species* (Table 12, Figure 19 and Figure 20). There was statistically insignificant ($P<0.05$) effect of negative control on the decline of the egg per gram of parasite load. The *Piperazine citrate* did not have any significant effect on the decline of parasite load especially Coccidia (Figure 20).

Piperazine is one of the ingredients in a number of combinations of anthehelminthic products. Piperazine is practically non toxic. The oral LD 50 for chicken is 8g/kg body weight. It can be used in animals of all ages. Piperazine paralyzes the worms, which are then eliminated by intestinal peristalsis. Piperazine also blocks the action of acetylcholine at the neuromuscular junctions of the worms (Georgi, 1980; Urquhart et al., 1996).

Coccidiostats are used to control coccidia related infections. The coccidiostatic activity of antiprotozoal drugs is related to its ability to competitively antagonize the physiological role of thiamine as a coenzyme (Georgi, 1980). This explains why *piperazine citrate* is not effective in the control of coccidia related infections (Figure 20).

On the other hand *Erythrina abyssinica* has important bioactive compounds namely tannins and anthraquinones. Tannins are produced to a greater or lesser degree by all plants. The harsh astringent taste of tannin laden bark and leaves makes them unpalatable to insects. Tannins draw the tissues closer together and improve their resistance to infection. Athraquinones are main active constituents in herbs. They have an irritant laxative effect on the large intestine causing contractions of the intestinal walls and stimulating bowel movements approximately 10 hours after being taken. They also make the stool more liquid, easing bowel movements and quick removal of paralyzed worms from the gut (Harbone, 1984). This explains why *Erythrina abyssinica* extracts are effective in the control of *Ascaridia galli* and *Trichostrongylus tenuis.*

As detailed in Table 13, neutrophils had normal physiological range values. Lymphocytes and Eosionphils were above normal values. Basophils, Red blood cells, haemoglobin had normal values. The MCV, MCH and MCHC had values above the normal range. In Table 14 it was shown that *alkaline phosphatase* was above normal values, *Alanine transaminase* and *Aspartate transaminase* were within normal ranges. Creatinine, Urease and Uric acid were slightly below than the normal expected values. Alkaline phosphatase (ALP) catalyzes the hydrolysis of phosphate esters in alkaline buffer and produces an organic radical and inorganic phosphate. Changes in alkaline phosphatase level and activity are associated with various disease states in the liver and bone (Abdi-Hachesco et al., 2011).

Conclusion and Recommendations

It can be concluded that *Erythrina abyssinica* was efficacious in the control of *Ascaridia galli.* It was also effective in the control of *Trychostrongylus tenuis* and coccidian parasites to a certain degree. Generally, haematological and biochemical tests reveal very minimum disturbances in the liver and kidney functions. It can therefore be concluded that, it is safe to use *Erythrina abyssinica* leaf extract in the control of *Ascaridia galli* infections, trychostronglids and coccidian parasites. Cases of reinfection for the case of coccidia are very common phenomena. The efficacy of *Erythrina abyssinica* is comparable to the conventional drug *Piperazine citrate. Piperazine citrate* is ineffective in the control of coccidia infections. The relationship between the treatment groups and egg per gram reduction was expressed in correlation rank coefficient (r^2). It ranged from *E. abyssinica leaves* extracts *(95.09%), (92.56%) Piperazine citrate* and (95.43%). negative control Further understanding of the bio active compounds responsible for activity against the parasites is vital.

It is also important to undertake sub acute and chronic toxicity studies. The study further recommends appropriate, simple and user friendly standardization of the extracts for farmers to use.

REFERENCES

Abdi-Hachesco B., Talebi. A and Asri-Rezaei Siamak (2011). Comparative Study on Blood Profiles of Indigenous and Ross-308 Broiler Breeders. *Global Veterinaria* 7 (3): 238-241, 2011.

Acamovic T., Sinurat A., Natarajan A., Anitha K., Chandrasekeran D., Shindey D., Sparks N., Oduguwa O., Mypeta B. and Kitalyi A. (2005). Poultry In: Livestock and Wealth creation, improving the husbandry of animals kept by resource-poor people in developing countries edited by Owen E, Kitalyi A, Jayasuriya N, and Smith T, Nottingham University Press, United Kingdom pp 303-313.

Adjanohou, J. E., Aboubakar, N., and Ebot, M.E. (1988). Traditional medicine and pharmacopeia contribution to ethno-botanical and floristic studies in Cameroon, CNPMS, Porto-Norvo, Benin.

Aerts, R.J., Barry, T.N., McNabb, W. C., 1999. Polyphenols and agriculture: beneficial effects of proanthocyanidins in forages. *Agricultural Ecosystems Environment,* 75: 1-12.

Agamemnon Despopoulos, M.D., Silbernagl M.D. (2003). Color Atlas of physiology 2003, Thieme ISBN 3-13-545003-8 (GTV).

Albokhadaim Ibrahim (2012). Hematological and some biochemical values of indigenous chickens in Al-Ahsa, Saudi Arabia during Summer Season. *Asian Journal of Poultry Science* 6 (4): 138-145, 2012 ISSN 189-3609/DOI: 10.3923/ajpsaj.138.145.

Alders R.G. and Pym R.A.E. (2009). Indigenous poultry: Still important to millions, eight thousand years after domestication. *World's Poultry Science Journal*, 65:181-190.

Alders R. G., Pym R.A.E. and Rushton J. (2009). Report on the Family Poultry Workshop held during the XXIII World's Poultry Congress. *World's Poultry Science Journal*, 65: 298-305.

Alders. R. and Spradbrow P. (2001) Controlling Newcastle Disease in Indigenous chickens. A field manual version 14.03.2001. Australian centre for Agricultural Research (ACIAR).

Alfred B., Msoffe P.L.M., Kajuna F.F., Bunn D., Muhairwa A.P. and Cardona C.J. (2012). Causes of losses in free range local chickens following control of Newcastle disease in three indigenouss in Morogoro, Tanzania. *Livestock Research for Rural Development. Volume 24, Article #124.* Retrieved November 8, 2012, from http://www.lrrd.org/ lrrd24/ 7/alfr24124.htm.

Allan,W.H., Gough, L.E. (1974). A standard haemaglutination inhibition test for Newcastle disease. A comparision of macro and micromethods. *Veterinary Research* 95: 120-123.

Ambrose P. (2005). Antimicrobial susceptibility break points. PKPD and susceptibility breakpoints. Treat Respiratory Medicine (Suppl 4) 1:5.

Athanasiadou S., Githiori J. and Kyriazakis I., (2007). Medicinal plants for Helminth parasite control: facts and fictions. *Animal.* 2007 Oct; 1(9):1392-400. Downloaded from the link; http://www.ncbi.nlm.nih.gov/ pubmed/22444894.

Athanasiadou, S., Kyriazakis, I., Jackson, F., Coop, R.L., (2001). Direct anthelmintic effects of condensed tannins towards different gastrointestinal nematodes of sheep: *Invitro* and *invivo* studies. *Veterinary Parasitology*, 99, 205–19.

Atsamo, A.D., Nguelefack, T.B., Datte, J.Y. and Kamanyi, A. (2011). Acute and subchronic oral toxicity assessment of the ethanolic extract from stem bark of *Erythrina senegalensis* DC (Fabaceae) in rodents. *J. Ethnopharmacology*. (2011).doi 10.1016/jep.2011.01.023.

Balakrishman V., Philip Robinson J., Manickasamy A., and Ravindran K C (2009). Ethno veterinary studies among farmers in Dindigul District Tamil Nadu, India. Global Journal of Pharmacology 3(1): 15-23, 2009. Retrieved from http://www.idosi.org/gjp/3(1)09/4.pdf

Banso A., Adeyemo S.O. (2007). Phytochemical and antimicrobial evaluation of ethanolic extract of *Dra-caena manni* Bark. *Nig. J.Biotech.* 18(1-2): 27-32.

Bate-Smith, E.C., 1962. The phenolic constituent of plants and their taxonomic significance, dicotyledons. J*ournal of the Linnean Society of London, Botany*, 58: 95–103.

Birdi T.J., Brijesh S., and Daswani P.G. (2006) "Approaches towards the preclinical testing and standardization of medicinal plants", *Foundation for Medicinal Research*, India, (2006).

Bizimenyera E.S., Swam G.E., Samdumu F.B., McGaw L.J. and Eloff J.N. (2007). Safety profiles of peltophorum africanum sond. (Fabaceae) extracts. PhD thesis, University of Pretoria, 2007: 67-78.

Branckaert R.D.S. (1996) From Backyard to Commercial Poultry production: The keys of success. Paper presented at an International Workshop on Newcastle disease, University of Pretoria, pp 9, Dec. 1996.

Brookes K.B., Katsoulis L.C. (2006). Bioactive components of *Rhoicissus tridentata*: a pregnancy-related traditional medicine. *South African Journal of Science*.102:267-272.

Bunalema L., Kirimuhuzya C., Tabuti J.R.S., Waako P., Magadula J.J., Otieno N., Orodho J.A., Okemo P., (2011). The efficacy of the crude root bark extracts of *Erythrina abyssinica* on Rifampicin Resistant *Mycobacterium tuberculosis*. Afr Health Sci. 11: 587–593.

Bussmann R.W., Malca G., Glenn A., Sharon D., Nilsen B., Parris B. , Dubose D., Ruiz D., Saleda J., Martinez M., Carillo L., Walker K., Kuhlman A., Townesmith (2011). Toxicity of medicinal plants used in traditional medicine in Northern Peru. *J. Ethnopharmacol.* 137(1):121-40.

Cenci F.B., Louvandini, H., McManus, C.M., DellPorto, A., Costa, D.M., Araújo, S.C., Minho, A.P., and Abdalla, A.L. (2007). Effects of condensed tannin from *Acacia mearnsii* on sheep infected naturally with gastrointestinal helminths. *Veterinary Parasitology*, Vol 144, issue 1-2,132-137.

Chacha M., Bojase-Moleta G. and Majinda R.T.R. (2004). Antimicrobial and radical scavenging flavonoids from the stem wood of *Erythrina latissima. Phytochemistry* Vol 66, Issue 1, pp 99-104.

Chinrasri Orawan and W. Aengwanich (2007). Blood Cell Characteristics, Hematological Values and Average Daily Gained Weight of Thai Indigenous, Thai Indigenous Crossbred and Broiler Chickens. *Pakistan Journal of Biological Sciences, 10: 302-309.*

Chandra P., Sachan N., Ghosh A.K. and Kishore K. (2010). Acute and Sub-chronic Oral Toxicity Studies of a Mineralo-herbal Drug Amlena on Experimental Rats. *International Journal of Pharmaceutical Research and Innovation*, Vol. 1: 15-18.

Djeraba, A., Quere, P. (2000). Invivo macrophage activation in chickens with acemannan, a complex carbohydrate extracted from Aloe vera. *International Journal of Immunology* 22: 365-372.

Donahue, M. J., Yacoub, N.J., Kaeini, M.R., Masaracchia, R.A., Harris, B.G., (1981). Glycogen metabolizing enzymes during starvation and feeding of

A. suum maintained in a perfusion chamber. *Journal of Parasitology*, 67: 505-510.

Ejobi, Mosha R.D., Ndege S. and Kamoga D. (2007). Ethno-veterinary medicinal plants of the Lake Victoria basin: A bioprospection. *Journal of Animal and Veterinary Advances* 6: 257-261. Retrieved from http://docsdrive.com/pdfs/medwelljournals/javaa/2007/257-261.pdf

Ejobi F. and Olila D. (2004). On-farm validation of selected ethno-veterinary medical practices in the Teso farming system. A technical report of NARO/DFID COARD. National Agriculture Research Organization. www.naro.go.ug/information/COARD

Ejobi, F., Mosha, R.D., Ndege, S., and Kamoga, D. (2007). Ethno-veterinary medicinal plants of the Lake Victoria basin: A bioprospection. *Journal of Animal and Veterinary Advances*, 6 (2): 257-261.

Fisher, R.A. and Yates, F. (1948). *Statistical tables for biological, agricultural and medical research* (3rd ed.). London: Oliver & Boyd. pp. 26–27

Food and Agriculture Organization (FAO 2001). The impact of HIV/AIDS on food security, Rome.

Gad, S.C., (2007). The Rat. In: Animal Models in Toxicology, Gad, S.C. (Ed.). CRC Press, Boca Raton, FL, ISBN: 10: 0824754077, pp: 193-195.

Gajendran K and Karthickeyan S.M.K. (2009). Status of indigenous ducks in Tamil Nadu, India: a traditional perspective. *Livestock Research for Rural Development. Volume 21, Article #175.* Retrieved November 8, 2012, from http://www.lrrd.org/lrrd21/10/gaje21175.htm

Gakuya D.W., (2001). Pharmacological and clinical evaluation of the anthelmintic activity of *Albizia anthelmintica* Brogn, *Maerua edulis* De wolf and *Maerua subcordata* De wolf plant extracts in sheep and mice. PhD thesis. University of Nairobi, Clinical Sciences Department; 2001.

Gbile, O.Z. (1991). Identification and pharmaceutical importance of medicinal plants. Ibadan: Forestry Research Institute of Nigeria, Ibadan, Nigeria.

GenStat (2011). GenStat 14th Edition. Lawes Agricultural Trust.

Georgi Jay R. (1980). Parasitology for Veterinarians. W. B Saunders Company, West Washington square, Philadelphia.

Ghosh, M.N. (1984). Fundamentals of Experimental Pharmacology. 2nd Edition. *Culcutta: Scientific Book Agency*; 1984. pp. 153–158.

Githiori J.B., (2004). Evaluation of anthelmintic properties of ethno veterinary plant preparations used as livestock dewormers by pastoralists and small holder farmers in Kenya. PhD thesis, Uppsala 2004. Acta Universitatis Agriculturae Sueciae Veterinaria 173.

Githiori J.B., Athanasiadou S., Thamsborg S.M.(2006). Use of plants in novel approaches for control of gastrointestinal helminths in livestock with emphasis on small ruminants. *Veterinary Parasitology*. 139(4):308–320.

Guéye E.F. (2009). The role of networks in information dissemination to family Poultry farmers, small- scale Family Poultry production, *Worlds Poultry Science Journal*, Vol 65, March, 2009 pp 115-124.

Gueye E.F. (2002). Newcastle disease in family poultry: prospects for its control through ethnoveterinary medicine. *Livestock Research for Rural Development* 14(5) 2002. Retrieved on November 8, 2012, from http://www.lrrd.org/lrrd14/5/guey145a.htm.

Hammond, J.A., Fielding, D. and Bishop, S.C., (1997). Prospects for plant anthelmintics in tropical veterinary medicine. *Veterinary Research Communications*, 21 (3), 213-228

Harbone J.B. (1984). Phytochemical methods. A guide to modern techniques of plant analysis. Chapman and Hall, London, United Kingdom.

Harborne, J. B. (1973). Phytochemical Methods. Chapman and Hall, London p. 113.

Haslwimmer. M. (1994). Is HIV/AIDS a threat to livestock production? The example of Rakai, Uganda. Retrieved from: http://www.fao.org/docrep/t4650t/t4650t17.htm

Hayes, A.W. (2007). Principles of Pathology for Toxicological Studies In: Principles and Methods of Toxicology, Hayes, A.W. (Ed.)., 5th Edn., CRC Press, New York, ISBN: 084933778X pp: 592.

Hodges J. (2009). Emerging boundaries for poultry production: challenges, dangers and opportunities. *World's Poultry Science Journal*, 65: 5-22.

Houghton B.A. & Raman A. (1988). Laboratory handbook for the fractionation of natual extracts, Chapman & Hall. London, pp 1-7.

Ichimaru, M., Moriyasu, M., Nishiyama, Y., Kato, A., Mathenge, S.G., Juma, F.D., & Nganga, J.N. (1996). Structural elucidation of new flavanones isolated from *Erythrina abyssinica*. *Journal of Natural Products*, Vol.59, No.12, pp. 1113-1116, ISSN 1520-6025

Igga, F.W. (2007). *In vitro* ant-helmintic activity of selected plants used in ethno-veterinary practices in Kabira sub-county, Rakai district. A Special Project Report. Makerere University.

Ikigai H., Nakae T., Hara Y., Shimamura T. (1993). Bacterial catechins damage the lipid bilayer. *Biochin. Biophys. Act*, 1147: 132-136.

Illango J., Etoori A., Olupot H. and Mabonga J. (2000). Rural poultry production in two agro-ecological zones. Proceedings of the Second Research Coordinating meeting on Family poultry production in

Africa. Morogoro, Tanzania, October, 2000 pp 118-136. IAEA http://www.iaea.org/nafa/d3/public/12-rural-illango.pdf

Illango J., Mukiibi-Muka G., Abila P. P., Musisi G. and Etoori A. (2008). The value of the Newcastle disease I-2 thermostable vaccine use in the rural free-range poultry management system in Uganda. *Volume 20, Article #145.* Retrieved November 8, 2012, from http://www.lrrd.org/lrrd20/9/illa20145.htm

ITDG and IIRR (1996). Ethno veterinary medicine in Kenya. Afield manual of traditional animal healthcare practices. Intermediate Technology Development Group (ITDG) and international Institute of rural reconstruction (IIRR), Nairobi, Kenya. ISBN 9966-9606-2-7.

Jensen H.A. (1996). Semi-scavenging model for rural poultry holding. Invited paper presented at the symposium on: Rural poultry development with focus on employment, income and role of women. Proceedings of XX World Poultry Congress, New Delhi, India, September 2-8, 1996, Volume 1. Retrieved from http://www.fao.org/docrep/004/AC150E/AC150E07.htm

Jordan F.T.W. and Pattison M. (1996). Enterobacteriaceae In: poultry diseases. W B Saunders Company Ltd London NW1 7 DX, India, Fourth Ed. pp 9-38.

Jordan J.W. and Alderson M. (2009). Scale, Skills and Sustainable livelihoods. Participatory approaches to improving poultry production in Peri-Urban communities, Evidence from South Africa. *Outlook on Agriculture* Vol 38, No 1, 2009 pp 83-88.

Joshua A.J., Goudar K.S., Sameera N., Pavan Kumar G., Murali B., Dinakar N. and Amit A. (2010). Safety Assessment of Herbal Formulations, Rumbion™ and Tyrel™ in Albino Wistar Rats. *American Journal of Pharmacology and Toxicology* 5 (1): 42-47, 2010 ISSN 1557-4962.

Kakeocha C. (1984). Pfizer Poultry Production handbook. Published by Pfizer Corporation, Nairobi in association with Macmillan education Ltd London and Oxford.

Katunguka-Rwakishaya, Nalule S.K. and Sabiiti E.N. (2004). Indigenous Knowledge in Ethno Veterinary Medicine in South Western Uganda. DHP Publications series No.9, March 2004, Dry land Husbandry Project (DHP).

Kitalyi A., Mtenga L., Moton J., McLeodi A., Thornton P., Dorward A. and Saadullah M. (2005). Why produce livestock if you are poor? In: Livestock and wealth creation. Improving the husbandry of animals kept by the resource-poor in developing countries, edited by Owen E; Kitalyi

A; Jayasuriya N and Smith T. 1stedition ISBN 1-904761-32-1 Nottingham University Press,United Kingdom.

Kitalyi, A.J. (1996). Socio-economic aspects of indigenous chicken production in Africa: the role of women, children and non-governmental organizations. Paper presented at the *XX World poultry Congress*, 2-5 September 1996, New Delhi.

Kitalyi, A.J. (1998). Indigenous chicken production systems in rural Africa. Household food security and gender issue, FAO Animal Production and Health Paper 142. Rome, Italy pp 160.

Kolawole O.D., Okorie V.O., Ogidiowa M.T. and Adeogun M.O. (2007). Ethno- Veterinary practices amongst small holder farmers in Ekiti state, Nigeria, *African Journal of traditional complimentary and alternative medicines* 4 (4): 443-468. Retrieved from http://www.bioline.org.br/ pdf?tc07061

Kotze, A. C., Clifford, S., O'Grady, J., Behnke, J. M. and McCarthy, J. S., (2004). An *in vitro* larval motility assay to determine anthelmintic sensitivity for human hookworm and *strongyloides* species. *American Journal of Tropical Medicine and Hygiene*. 71(5):608-16.

Lagu C. and Kayanja F.I.B. (2010): Medicinal plant extracts widely used in the control of Newcastle disease (NCD) and helminthosis among indigenous chickens of South Western Uganda. *Livestock Research for Rural Development. Volume 22, Article #200.* Retrieved November 2, 2011, from http://www.lrrd.org/lrrd22/11/lagu22200.htm

Lagu C., Mugisha A. and Koma L.M.P.K. 2011: Impact of HIV/AIDS on the Livestock-Producing Communities of Uganda: Case Studies of Moyo and Kashumba Sub counties. *Livestock Research for Rural Development.* Volume 23, Article #123. Retrieved March 16, 2012, from http://www.lrrd.org/lrrd23/6/lagu23123.htm

Lagu C. and Kayanja Frederick I.B. (2013b). Acute Toxicity Profiles of Aqueous and Ethanolic Extracts of Capsicum annum Seeds from South Western Uganda, Insights from Veterinary Medicine, Dr. Rita Payan Carreira (Ed.), ISBN: 978-953-51-1005-7, InTech, DOI: 10.5772/53599. Available from: http://www.intechopen.com/books/insights-from-veterinary-medicine/acute-toxicity-profiles-of-aqueous-and-ethanolic-extracts-of-capsicum-annum-seeds-from-south-western

Lagu C. and Kayanja F.I.B. (2013a). The invitro Antihelminthic Efficacy of *Erythrina Abyssinica* Extracts on Ascaridia galli, Insights from Veterinary Medicine, Dr. Rita Payan Carreira (Ed.), ISBN: 978-953-51-1005-7, InTech, DOI: 10.5772/53708. Available from:

http://www.intechopen.com/books/insights-from-veterinary-medicine/the-in-vitro-antihelminthic-efficacy-of-erythrina-abyssinica-extracts-on-ascaridia-galli.

Lagu C. and Kayanja I.B. Frederick (2012). Invitro Antimicrobial Activity of Crude Extracts of *Erythrina abyssinica* and *Capsicum annum* in Poultry Diseases Control in the South Western Agro-Ecological Zone of Uganda, A Bird's-Eye View of Veterinary Medicine, Carlos C. Perez-Marin (Ed.), ISBN: 978-953-51-0031-7, InTech, Available from: http://www.intechopen.com/articles/show/title/in-vitro-antimicrobial-activity-of-crude-extracts-of-erythrina-abyssinica-and-capsicum-annum-in-poul

Nalule A.S, Mbaria J.M, Kimenju J.W and Olila D. (2012): Ascaricidal activity of *Rhoicissus tridentata* root-tuber ethanolic and water extracts. *Livestock Research for Rural Development. Volume 24, Article #144.* Retrieved September 4, 2012, from http://www.lrrd.org/lrrd24/8/ nalu24144.htm.

Li Hui, Ramon F. Thali, Christy Smolak, Fan Gong, Rodrigo Alzamora, Theo Wallimann, Roland Scholz, Núria M. Pastor-Soler, Dietbert Neumann,and Kenneth R. Hallows (2010). Regulation of the creatine transporter by AMP-activated protein kinase in kidney epithelial cells. *American Journal of Physiology Renal Physiology*. 2010 July; 299(1): F167–F177.

MAAIF (Ministry of Agriculture Animal Industry and Fisheries) and UBOS (Uganda Bureau of statistics) (2008). The National Livestock census. A summary report of the National Livestock Census, 2008.

Malu S.P., Obochi G.O., Edem C.A., Nyong B.E. (2009). Effect of methods of extraction on phytochemical constituents and antibacterial properties of *Tetracarpidium conophorum* seeds, *Global Journal of Pure and Applied Sciences*. 15: 373-376.

Marcus, S. (1992). A preliminary study on the anthelmintic properties of *Terminalia glaucescens* in cattle in Northwest province of Cameroon: An ethno-veterinarian approach. DVM Thesis. Utrecht: University of Utrecht, Faculty of Veterinary Medicine.

Masimba E.S., Mbiriri D.T., Kashangura M.T. and Mutibvu T. (2011). Indigenous practices for the control and treatment of ailments in Zimbabwe's indigenous poultry. *Livestock Research for Rural Development. Volume 23, Article #257.* Retrieved September 4, 2012, from http://www.lrrd.org/lrrd23/12/masi23257.htm

Masola, S.N., Mosha, R.D., Wambura, P.N. (2009). Assessment of antibacterial activity of crude extracts of stem and root barks from

Adansonia digitata (Bombacaceae) (African baobab). *African Journal of Biotechnology* Vol.8 (19), pp 5076-5083. ISSN 1684-5315, Academic Journals.

Mathias, E., Rangnekar, D.V. and McCorkle, C.M. (1999). Ethno veterinary Medicine: Alternatives for Livestock Development. Proceedings of an International Conference held in Pune, India, on November 4-6, 1997. Volume 1: Selected Papers. BAIF Development Research Foundation, Pune, India.

McCorkle, C.M. (1986). An introduction to Ethnoveterinary Research and Development. *Journal of Ethnobiology* 6 (1): 129-149.

Meng. Q., Niu Yu., Niu Xiwu., Roubin R.H., Hanrahan J.R. (2009). Ethnobotany, Phytochemistry and pharmacology of the genus Caragana used in traditional Chinese medicine. *Journal of Ethno pharmacology* 124: 350-368.

Min, B.R., Barry, T.N., Attwood, G.T., and McNabb, W.C. (2003). The effect of condensed tannins on the nutrition and health of ruminants fed fresh temperate forages: a review. *Animal Feed Science and Technology*, 106: 3–19.

Ministry of Agriculture, Animal Industry and Fisheries (MAAIF 2000). Agricultural Response to HIV/AIDS epidemic. A paper presentation at imperial botanical beach hotel, Entebbe.

Mojab F, Kamalinejad M, Ghaderi N, Vahidipour H. R (2003). Phytochemical Screening of Some Species of Iranian Plants. *Iranian Journal of Pharmaceutical Research* (2003), 77-82.

Molan, A.L., Waghorn, G.C., Min, B.R. and McNabb, W.C., (2000).The effect of condensed tannins from seven herbages of *Trichostrongylus columbriformis* larval migration in vitro. *Folia Parasitological*, 47: 39-44.

Monjanel-Mouterde S., Traore F., Gasquet M., Dodero F., Delmas F., Ikoli J. F., Lorec A.M., Chamlian V., Portugal H., Balansard G and Pisano P (2006). Lack of toxicity of hydroethanolic extracts Mitragyna inermis (Willd.) O. Kuntze by gavage in the rat. *Journal of Ethnopharmacology,* 103(3):319-26.

Morgan D.W. and Krejcie R.V. (1970). Determining sample size for research activities, Educational and Psychological measurement, 30, 608, Sage publications. Retrieved from http://www. sageperformance.com/ drjeffallen/DrA/Teaching/5480/samplesize.htm.

Moriyasu, M., Ichimaru, M., Nishiyama, Y., Kato, A., Mathenge, G.S., Juma, F.D., & Nganga, J.N. (1998). Minor flavanones from *Erythrina abyssinica*. *Journal of Natural Products*, 61, 185–188.

Mtambo. M.M.A., Mushi E.J., Kinabo L.D.B., Maeda-Machang'u A., Mwamengele G.L.M., Yongolo M.G.S. and Temu R.P.C. (1999). Evaluation of the efficacy of the crude extracts of *Capsicum frutescens, Citrus limon* and *Opuntia vulgaris* against Newcastle disease in domestic fowl in Tanzania. Elsevier Science Ireland Ltd.

Mwakapuja R.S., Msoffe P.L.M., Kajuna F., Bunn D. and Cardona C.J. (2012). Newcastle disease virus immunization with I-2 vaccine: a case study of local free range chickens in rural communities in Morogoro, Tanzania. *Livestock Research for Rural Development. Volume 24, Article #123.* Retrieved November 8, 2012, from http://www.lrrd.org/lrrd24/7/ nwak24123.htm.

NAADS (National Agricultural Advisory Services) (2003). Baseline report on the agricultural sector and rural livelihoods in Uganda.

Naido, V., (2005). Screening of four major plants commonly used in ethno veterinary medicine for antimicrobial and protozoal and antioxidant activity. Unpublished Master of Science thesis, University of Pretoria Ltd.

Nalule A.S., Mbaria J.M., Olila D. and Kimenju J.W. (2011). Ethnopharmacological practices in management of livestock helminths by pastoral communities in the drylands of Uganda. *Livestock Research for Rural Development. Volume 23, Article #36.*Retrieved May 18, 2011, from http://www.lrrd.org/lrrd23/2/nalu23036.htm.

Nanyingi. M.O., Mbaria J.M., Lanyasunya, A.L., Wagate, C.G ., Koros, K.B., Kaburia, H.F., Munenge. R.W. and Ogara W.O. (2008). Ethnopharmacological survey of Samburu district, Kenya. *Journal of Ethnobiology and Ethnomedicine*. 4:14.

National Council (1991). Micro livestock: Little-Known small animals with a promising economic future. National academy press, Washington, D.C.

Nowaczewski and Kontecka (2011). Haematological indices, size of erythrocytes and haemoglobin saturation in broiler chickens kept in commercial conditions. *Animal Science Papers and Reports* vol. 30 (2012), no. 2, 181-190 Institute of Genetics and Animal Breeding, Jastrzębiec, Poland.

Nsubuga-Mutaka R., Ssenteza J. and Niwagaba B. (2005). Livestock Indigenous Technical Knowledge, *Mbarara zonal Agriculture Research and Development Institute book Part 1,* Volume 1.Unpublished report.

Nuwanyakpa, M., DeVeries, J., Ndi, C and Django, S. (1990). Traditional veterinary medicine in Cameroon: A renaissance in an ancient indigenous technology. Bamenda: HPI, Cameroon.

Nuwanyakpa, M., Django, S., Toyang, J. Ndi, C. and Ndi, A. (1995). Animal healthcare and para-veterinary medicine in the North-western province in Cameroon. *Proceedings of an Ethnovet Workshop*, Sagba: HPI, Cameroon.

O.I.E (1996). The Newcastle disease. In: Manual of standards for diagnostic Tests and vaccines, pp 161-169.

O'Hara M., Kiefer D., Farrel K., Kemper K. (1998). A review of 12 commonly used medicinal herbs. *Arch. Fam. Med.* 7(6):523-36.

Ogundare A.O., Adetuyi F.C., Akinyosoye F.A. (2006). Antimicrobial activity of *Vernonia tenoreana*. *Afr.J. Biotech.*5 (18):1663-1668.

Okigbo R.N., Eme U.E., Ogbogu S. (2008). Biodiversity and conservation of medicinal and aromatic plants in Africa. *Biotechnol. Mol. Biol. Rev.*3(6): 127-134.

Okitoi L.O., Ondwasy H.O., Siamba D.N. and Nkurumah D. (2007). Traditional herbal preparations for indigenous poultry health management in Western Kenya. *Livestock Research for Rural Development.* Volume 19, Article #72. Retrieved June 30, 2010, from http://www.lrrd.org/lrrd19/5/okit19072.htm

Olila D., Bukenya-Ziraba R. and Kamoga D. (2007). Bio-prospective studies on medicinal plants used to manage poultry diseases in the Mount Elgon region of Uganda. *Research Journal of Pharmacology* 1: 56-60.retrieved from http://docsdrive.com/pdfs/medwelljournals/rjpharm/2007/56-60.pdf

Olila, D. and Bukenya, R. (2005). A survey of medicinal plants used for treating poultry diseases in eastern and central Uganda. A Technical Project Report. Unpublished Report.

Olivier A. (2004). Newcastle disease. Department: Agriculture Republic of South Africa http://www.nda.agric.za/docs/Infopaks/Newcastle.pdf

Organization for Economic Co-operation and Development (OECD), (1995). Guidelines for the Testing of Chemicals (No. 407, Section 4: Health Effects) "Repeated Dose 28-Day Oral Toxicity in Rodents" (Adopted on 12 May 198 1 and Updated on 27 July 1995.).

Organization for Economic Co-operation and Development, 2000. Guidance document on the recognition, assessment and use of clinical signs as humane endpoints for experimental animals used in safety evaluation. Environmental Health and Safety Monograph Series on Testing and Assessment No.

Petrus N.P., Mpofu I. and Lutaaya E. (2011). The care and management of indigenous chicken in Northern communal areas of Namibia. *Livestock*

Research for Rural Development. Volume 23, Article #253. Retrieved November 8, 2012, from http://www.lrrd.org/lrrd23/12/petr23253.htm.

Ramdas,S.R. 2009. Reclaiming endangered livelihoods: untold stories of indigenous women and backyard poultry. *World's Poultry Science Journal.* 65: 241-249.

Satrija, F., Nansen, P., Murtini, S., and He, S. (1995). Anthelmintic activity of papaya latex against patent *Heligmosomoides polygrus* infection in mice. *Journal of Ethnopharmacology,* 48:161-164.

Schmincke K.H. (2003). Medicinal Plants for forest conservation and healthcare. Non-Wood Forest Products 11, Food and Agriculture Organization of the United Nations.

Schoenian, S. (2008). Understanding anthelmintics (dewormers). Small Ruminant Info Series. Western Maryland Research & Education Center, University of Maryland Cooperative Extension.

Sharmin M.L. and Myenuddin M. (2004). Hematological values of the indigenous chickens. *Bangl. J. Vet Med.* (2004). 2 (2): 163-164.

Simaraks, S., Chinrasri .O. and Aengwanich (2004). Hematological, electrolyte and serum biochemical vakue of the Thai indigenous (Gallus domesticus) in northeastern of Thailand. *Songklanakarin J. Science and Technol.* 26: 425-430.

Smith E.M. and Hattingh J. (1979). The Lability of some haematological parameters in chickens and ducks. *S. Afr. J Anim. Sci.* 9:11-15 (1979).

Soetan K.O. and Aiyelaagbe O.O. (2009). The need for bioactivity-safety evaluation and conservation of medicinal plants - A review. *Journal of Medicinal Plants Research* Vol. 3(5): 324-328, Available online at http://www.academicjournals.org/JMPR.

Spradbrow, P.B. (1993-94). Newcastle disease in indigenous chickens. *Poultry Science Review* 5: 57-96.

Street R.A., Stirk W.A. and Van Staden J. (2008). South African traditional medicinal Plant trade-Challenges in regulating quality, safety and efficacy. *Journal of Ethno pharmacology* 119: 705-710.

Tadelle D. (1996). Studies on indigenous poultry production systems in the Central Highlands of Ethiopia. Swedish University of Agricultural Science. (M.Sc. thesis).

Tadelle D. and Ogle B. (2001). Indigenous Poultry Production systems in Central highlands of Ethiopia. *Tropical Animal Health and Production* 33(6): 521-537.

Thompson, D.P. and Geary, T.G., (1995). The structure and function of helminth surfaces. In: Marr J.J, (Edn). Biochemistry and Molecular Biology of Parasites. 1st Ed. New York: Academic Press 203–32.

Thrusfield, M. (2003). Veterinary Epidemiology. Blackwell Publishing, Berlin Germany

Tolossa Y.H., Shafi Z.D. and Basu A.K. (2009). Ectoparasites and gastrointestinal helminths of chickens of three agro-climatic zones in Oromia Region, Ethiopia. *Animal Biology* 59: 289-297.

UBOS (Uganda Bureau of statistics) (2004). Report on the agricultural module, piggy-backed onto the population and housing census (PHC), 2002. Household based agricultural activities, crop livestock and poultry characteristics pp 47-49.

UBOS (Uganda Bureau of statistics) (2006). Uganda national household survey, Socio-economic module 2005-2006, Entebbe, Uganda.

UBOS (Uganda Bureau of statistics) (2009). Statistical abstract.

UNESCO (1996). Culture and Health, Orientation texts- World Decade for Cultural Development Documents CLT/DEC. PRO-1996, Paris, France, p. 29.

Urquhart G.M., Armour J., Duncan J.L., Dunn A.M. and Jennings F.W. (1996). Veterinary Parasitology. *Blackwell Publishing Company* pp 10-137.

Waghorn, G.C., and McNabb, W.C. (2003). Consequences of plant phenolic compounds for productivity and health of ruminants. Proceedings of the Nutrition Society, 62, 383–392.

Waihenya R.K., Mtambo M.M.A. and Nkwengulila G. (2002). Evaluation of the efficacy of the crude extract of *Aloe secundiflora* in chickens experimentally infected with Newcastle disease virus. *Journal of Ethnopharmacology* 79: 299-304.

Walker D. Robert (2006). Antimicrobial susceptibility testing methods and interpretation of results In: Antimicrobial therapy in Veterinary Medicine, Fourth Edition, *Blackwell publishing* pp11-25, Iowa State University, USA.

Wang Cuina, Zhang Tiehua, Liu Jun, Lu Shuang, Zhang Cheng, Wang Erlei, Wang Zuozhao, Zhang Yan, Liu Jingbo (2011). Subchronic toxicity study of corn silk with rats. *Journal of ethnopharmacology.* 137(1), 36-43.

Wanzala W., Zessin K.H., Kyule N.M., Baumann M.P.O., Mathias E. and Hassanali A. (2005): Ethnoveterinary medicine: a critical review of its evolution, perception, understanding and the way forward. *Livestock*

Research for Rural Development. Volume 17, Article #119. Retrieved August 1, 2014, from http://www.lrrd.org/lrrd17/11/wanz17119.htm

Wasswa P. and Olila D. (2006). The *in-vitro* Ascaricidal activity of selected indigenous medicinal plants used in Ethno Veterinary practices in Uganda. *African Journal of Traditional, Complementary and Alternative Medicines* 3, No. 2, (94-103)

Wofgang, K. and Sollod, A. (1986). Traditional veterinary medical practice by the Tuareg herders in Central Niger. Intergrated Livestock project, Ministry of Animal Resources, Niger.

Wong-Leung, V.L. (1988). Anti-microbial activities of some Hong Kong plants used in Chinese medicine. *Fitoterapia,* 59:11-16.

Yongolo, M.G.S., (1996). Epidemiology of Newcastle disease virus in indigenous chickens in Tanzania. MVM Dissertation, Sokoine University of Agriculture, Tanzania pp. 230.

Zieger U. *Veterinary Clinical Pathology*. Laboratory manual.

APPENDICES

Mbarara University of Science and Technology
Questionnaire for PhD Study

APPENDIX 1: ETHNO VETERINARY USES FOR CONTROL OF NEWCASTLE DISEASE AND HELMINTHOSIS AMONG INDIGENOUS CHICKENS IN THE SOUTH WESTERN AGRO ECOLOGICAL ZONE (SWAEZ) OF UGANDA

Questionnaire for Free range Poultry Farmers, traditional healers and users of poultry Indigenous technical knowledge's.

Introductions

Dear respondent, this questionnaire is contributing to the research entitled "Assessment of ethno veterinary practices in the management of Newcastle Disease and Helminthosis among Indigenous Chickens in the South Western Agro Ecological Zone (SWAEZ) of Uganda".

The information generated here shall be used as a baseline for further scientific research in the cost effective control measures of NCD and Helminthosis among indigenous chicken in the SWAEZ. Your responses will be treated confidentially. So I encourage you to be free and give us correct information as much as possible.

Thank you very much

Respondent's socio-economic data

1.0. District .... 2.0. Sub county.......................
3.0. Parish .... 4.0. Indigenous ....
5.0. Name of Recorder...................... 6.0. Date ....
6.0. Occupation of person being interviewed ....
7.0. Name of respondent (optional).........Sex ....
8.0. Name of the interviewer ....
9.0. Location ....

Specifics

10.0. Experience in poultry keeping .... (years)..............date
11.0. Which types of poultry do you keep?

Poultry species	Numbers
Indigenous chickens	
Commercial Layers	
Commercial broilers	
Ducks	
Turkeys	

12.0. What types of management practices do you practice?

Systems of Management	Description
Housing	
Feeding	
Watering	
Supplementation	
Deworming	
Vaccinations	
Prophylaxis	
Prevention against vermin's	

13.0. What common diseases are you facing in your flock?

Local Names	Scientific name	Clinical signs	Seasonality	Mode of spread

14. What traditional methods do you use for treating common diseases of poultry?

No	Health problems	Ingredient/ Quality used	Preparation and method of administration	Dosage	Level of confidence

Key for confidence level. 1. High 2. Medium 3. Low

15. How do you know that traditional medicines are effective?

1. Full Recovery 2. Partial recovery 3. Symptomatic recovery

16. Besides the traditional Veterinary Medicine (TVM), do you use the most recent Veterinary medicine? (1984)

17. If yes when do you prefer to use modern Veterinary practices?

a. When TVM does not show sign of improvement
b. For Vaccination
c. When TVM is not known
d. Others (Specify)...

18. Why do you combine traditional and modern Veterinary Medicine (MVM) in the management of poultry diseases?

Reasons:

....
....
....

19. What are the advantages of using TVM over that of MVM in poultry disease management?

Advantages	**Disadvantages**
1.	1.
2.	2.
3.	3.
4.	4.

20. Is there any Government Veterinarian or Animal health assistant coming to treat your poultry from related diseases?

1. Yes	
2. No	

21. If yes what problems do you encounter using Government Veterinary Services?

Reasons:

a. ....

b. ....

c. ....

d. ....

e. ....

22. Do you have traditional healers?

1. Yes	
2. No	

23. Have you ever taken your chickens to traditional healers for treatment?

1. Yes	
2. No	

24. How do they treat the chickens?

a..

b..

c..

d..

25. Are the treatments successful?

1. Yes	
2. No	

26. Are the Government Veterinary Services efficient?

1. Agree	
2. Strongly Agree	
3. Disagree	
4.Strongly Disagree	

27. What do you recommend should be done to improve the utilization of ethno Veterinary practices in poultry disease management?

a...

b...

c...

d...

APPENDIX 2: ETHNO VETERINARY USES FOR CONTROL OF NEWCASTLE DISEASE AND HELMINTHOSIS AMONG INDIGENOUS CHICKENS IN IHE SOUTH WESTERN AGRO ECOLOGICAL ZONE (SWAEZ) OF UGANDA

Questionnaire for Veterinarians/ Animal health assistants/ key informants

INTRODUCTIONS

Dear respondent, this questionnaire is contributing to the research entitled "Assessment of ethno veterinary practices in the management of Newcastle Disease and Helminthosis among Indigenous Chickens in the South Western Agro Ecological Zone (SWAEZ) of Uganda''.

The information generated here shall be used as a baseline for further scientific research in the cost effective control measures of NCD and Helminthosis among indigenous chicken in the SWAEZ. Your responses will be treated confidentially. So I encourage you to be free and give us correct information as much as possible.

Thank you very much

Respondent's socio-economic data

1.0. District .... 2.0. Sub county........................

3.0. Parish .... 4.0. Indigenous ....

5.0. Name of Recorder........................ 6.0. Date ....

6.0. Sex of the interviewee ....

7.0. Name of Veterinarian/ Animal health assistant ....
8.0. Job Position ....
9.0. Qualification ....
8.0. Name of the interviewer ....
9.0. Location ....
10.0. Experience in treating poultry .... (Years)...................... ......

Specifics

11. Do you offer Veterinary services to poultry farmers?

1. Yes	
2. No	

12. What types of poultry do you treat most frequently?

Poultry species	Numbers
Indigenous chickens	
Commercial Layers	
Commercial broilers	
Ducks	
Turkeys	
Others (specify)	

13. How often do you provide veterinary service?

1. Once in a week	
2. Once in two weeks	
3. Once in three weeks	
4. Once a month	
5. Others (specify)	

14. What transport do you use to reach your poultry farmers?
15. Do charge for Veterinary Services or it is offered free?

1. Free	
2. Sometimes i charge	
3. Sometimes I charge	
4. I never charge	
5. Others (specify)	

16. What problems prevent you from offering more efficient veterinary services?

a...

b...

c...

d...

Veterinary services, what do they do to their sick birds?

1. Treat	
2. Do nothing	
3. I do not know	
4. Others (specify)	

18. If they treat what Veterinary medicine do they normally use?

1. Ethno veterinary medicine	
2. Modern medicine	
3. Others (specify)	

19. Do you use traditional medicine while rendering your service?

1. Yes	
2. No	

20. If yes what makes you use traditional medicine?

....

....

....

....

....

21. if NO what makes you not use traditional medicine?
……………………………………………………………………………………
……………………………………………………………………………………
……………………………………………………………………………………
……………………………………………………………………………………

22. Which traditional medicines are most effective in the management of NCD and Helminthosis?

a.……………………………………………………………………………
b. …………………………………………………………………………
c.……………………………………………………………………………
d.……………………………………………………………………………
e.……………………………………………………………………………
f.……………………………………………………………………………
g.……………………………………………………………………………
h.……………………………………………………………………………

23. How do you use the above medicines? Give details of each?

a	
b	
c	
d	
e	
f	
g	
h	

24. Where did you learn to use traditional medicine? ....

25. What are the advantages of using traditional Veterinary Medicine (TVM) over that of Conventional Modern Veterinary Medicine (MVM) in poultry disease management?

Advantages	**Disadvantages**
5.	1.
6.	2.
7.	3.
8.	4.

26. Are your activities demand driven?

1. Yes	
2. No	

27. What problems do face if any while delivering Veterinary services to poultry farmers?

a..
b..
c...
d...

28. What problems do you face from Veterinary Government office while offering your services?

a..
b..

29. What is the scope for integrating traditional and modern Veterinary services?

....
....
....
....
....
....

30. What development would like to see happen over the next 5-10 years in Uganda?

a ....
b ....
c ....
d ....

31. Any specific comments you would like to talk about?

PROBIT CONVERSION TABLES

%	0	1	2	3	4	5	6	7	8	9
0		2.67	2.95	3.12	3.25	3.36	3.45	3.52	3.59	3.66
10	3.72	3.77	3.82	3.87	3.92	3.96	4.01	4.05	4.08	4.12
20	4.16	4.19	4.23	4.26	4.29	4.33	4.36	4.39	4.42	4.45
30	4.48	4.50	4.53	4.56	4.49	4.61	4.64	4.67	4.69	4.72
40	4.75	4.77	4.80	4.82	4.85	4.87	4.90	4.92	4.95	4.97
50	5.00	5.03	5.05	5.08	5.10	5.13	5.15	5.18	5.20	5.23
60	5.25	5.28	5.31	5.33	5.36	5.39	5.41	5.44	5.47	5.50
70	5.52	5.55	5.58	5.61	5.64	5.67	5.71	5.74	5.77	5.81
80	5.84	5.88	5.92	5.95	5.99	6.04	6.08	6.13	6.18	6.23
90	6.28	6.34	6.41	6.48	6.55	6.64	6.75	6.88	7.05	7.33

Source: Ghosh MN (1984); Fundamentals of Experimental Pharmacology

The percentage dead for 0 and 100 will be corrected before determination of LD50 using the formula (Ghosh (1984) shown below. *For 0%dead : 100(0.25/n); For 100%dead: 100(n-0.25/n).*

PICTURES OF VARIOUS MATERIALS AND PROCUDURES

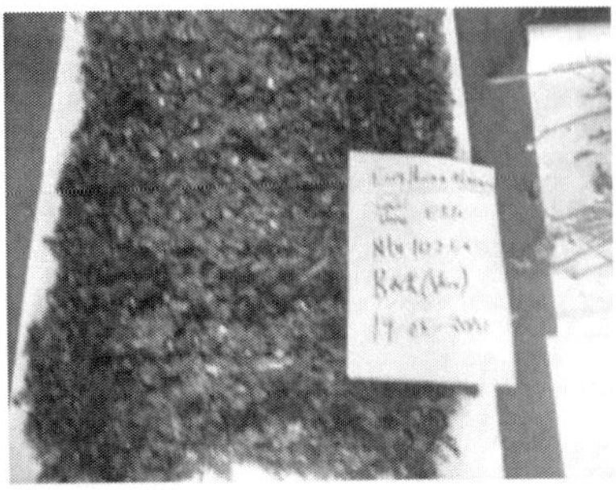

(a) Drying stem bark of *Erythrina abyssinica*

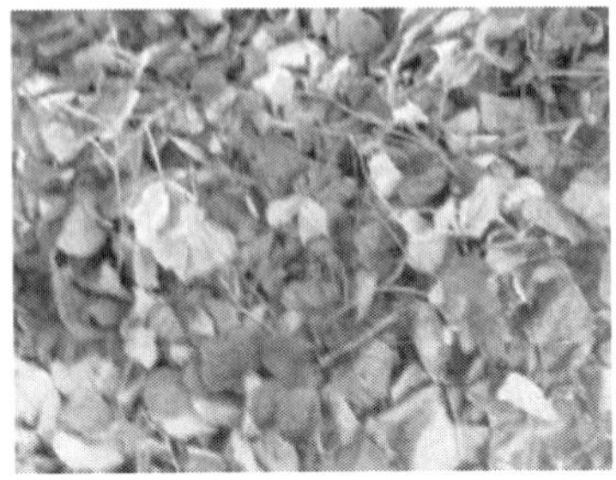

(b) Leaves of *Erythrina abyssinica*

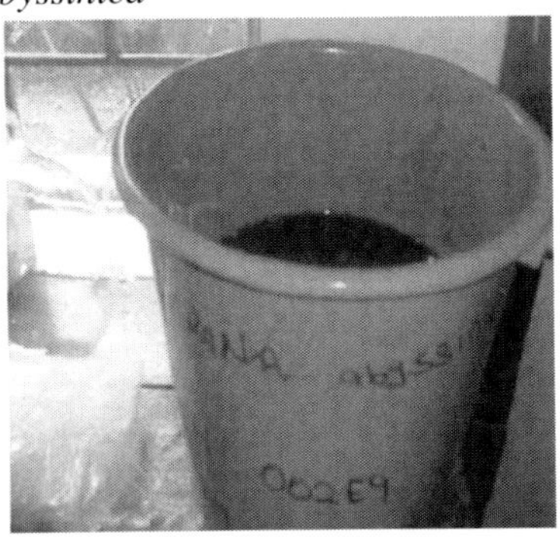

(c) Extracts of *Erythrina abyssinica*

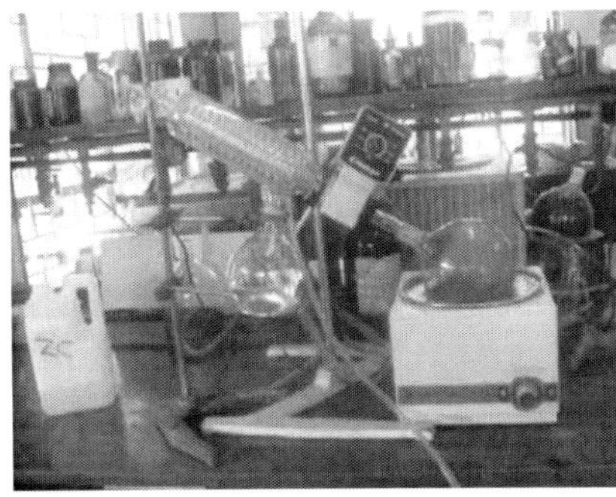

(d) Concentration of Extracts using Rotary evaporator

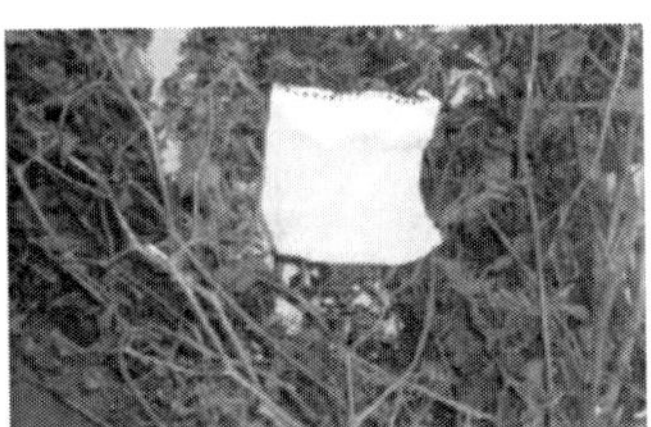

(e) Leaves and Fruits of *Capsicum annum* being dried

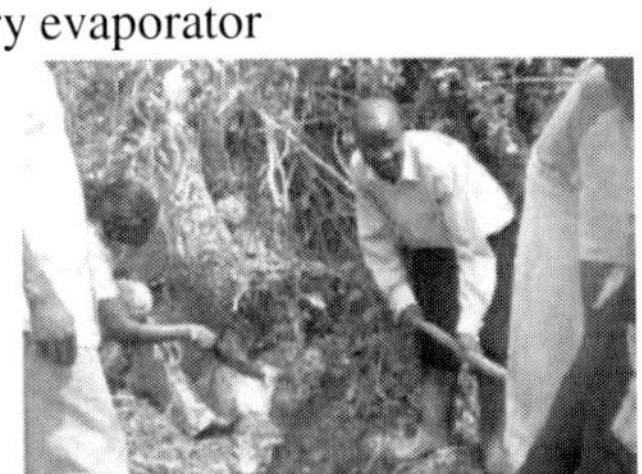

(f) Harvesting of Rootbark of *Erythrina abyssinica*

INDEX

C

D

M

N

O

P

Q

R

S

T

U

V

W

Y

Z